THE KETO RESET DIET
COOKBOOK

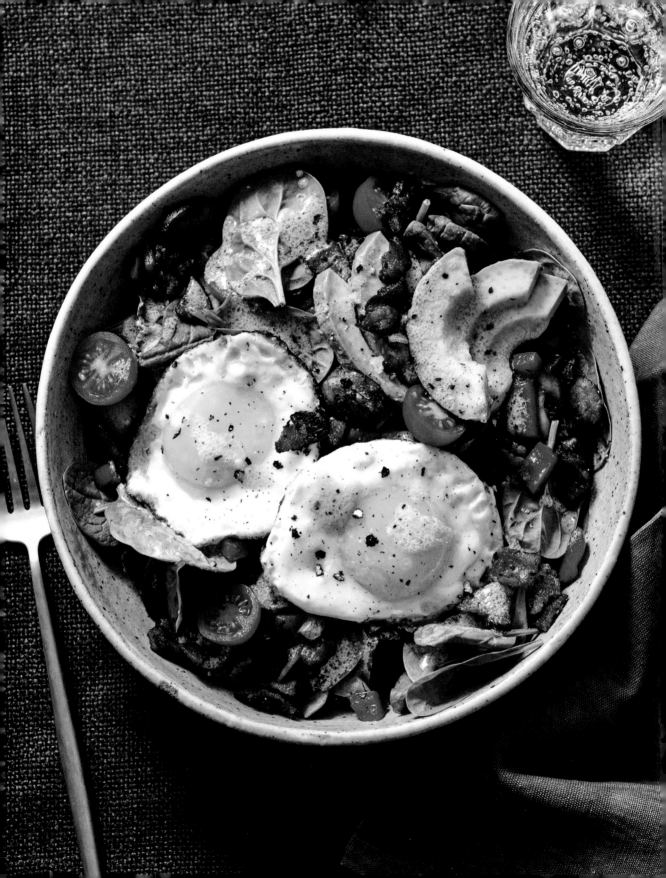

150 LOW-CARB, HIGH-FAT **KETOGENIC** RECIPES TO BOOST WEIGHT LOSS

THE KETO RESET DIET COOKBOOK

MARK SISSON WITH LINDSAY TAYLOR, PhD

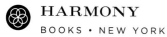

HARMONY
BOOKS · NEW YORK

The material in this book is for informational purposes only and is not intended as a substitute for the advice and care of your physician. As with all new diet and nutrition regimens, the program described in this book should be followed only after first consulting with your physician to make sure it is appropriate to your individual circumstances. The author and publisher expressly disclaim responsibility for any adverse effects that may result from the use or application of the information contained in this book.

Published in the United States by Harmony Books, an imprint of the Crown Publishing Group, a division of Penguin Random House LLC, New York.
crownpublishing.com

Harmony Books is a registered trademark, and the Circle colophon is a trademark of Penguin Random House LLC.

Library of Congress Cataloging-in-Publication Data
Names: Sisson, Mark, 1953– author. | Taylor, Lindsay, PhD, author.
Title: The keto reset diet cookbook: 150 low-carb, high-fat ketogenic recipes to boost weight loss / Mark Sisson and Lindsay Taylor, PhD
Description: New York: Harmony, 2018. | Includes index.
Identifiers: LCCN 2018020971 | ISBN 9780525576761 (hardcover) | ISBN 9780525576778 (ebook)
Subjects: LCSH: Reducing diets—Recipes. | Ketogenic diet—Recipes. | BISAC: HEALTH & FITNESS / Diets. | COOKING / Health & Healing / General. | COOKING / Health & Healing / Low Carbohydrate. | LCGFT: Cookbooks.
Classification: LCC RM222.2 .S5582 2018 | DDC 641.5/63—dc23 LC record available at https://lccn.loc.gov/2018020971.

ISBN 978-0-525-57676-1
Ebook ISBN 978-0-525-57677-8

Printed in the United States of America

Book and cover design by Jennifer K. Beal Davis
Jacket photographs by Andrew Purcell

10 9 8 7 6 5 4 3 2 1

First Edition

This book is dedicated to keto enthusiasts everywhere, who show tremendous curiosity and devotion to being as healthy as possible—even when cultural forces and conventional dietary wisdom are against them. It has been a long journey from the humble beginnings of my MarksDailyApple.com blog, talking about how a grain-based diet might be bad for you, to today's widespread acceptance of ancestral-style eating—and now the exploration of the highest level of sophistication of ancestral eating with keto. I have learned so much along the way, especially from the experiences and authentic feedback of members of the primal and keto community. I have been profoundly touched by the thousands of letters, photographs, and personal interactions I've had with people who have transformed their lives. The message you receive today in my books and multimedia educational programs about optimal health practices and dietary particulars is indeed the result of a group effort, for your inspiration is what keeps me going day after day without a second thought. Keep up the devoted effort, and live awesome!

CONTENTS

INTRODUCTION

The opportunity to share these wonderful keto-friendly recipes with you comes from the success of *The Keto Reset Diet*, released in October 2017. That book delivered a comprehensive education on the benefits of nutritional ketosis along with practical steps to go keto the right way, avoiding the risks of backsliding and burnout that happen when you attempt dietary transformation with a flawed approach. With the book well-received and the keto movement becoming increasingly popular, many people have asked me for more help with the day-to-day planning of meals to make keto easy, interesting, and varied. In May of 2018, I released an entire book dedicated to keto recipes for the Instant Pot multiuse electric pressure cooker: *The Keto Reset Instant Pot Cookbook* (written with Lindsay Taylor and Layla McGowan). I called that book the ultimate in efficiency—both time efficient with the Instant Pot and metabolically efficient when you hone your keto skills! I have also been working feverishly with my coauthor, Lindsay, and other members of the team at my Primal Kitchen company since the release of *The Keto Reset Diet* to create, test, and perfect a broad selection of keto-friendly recipes.

This *Keto Reset Diet Cookbook* is the result of that effort. We designed it to offer something for every keto enthusiast. If you are pressed for time and not highly competent in the kitchen, you'll find simple, go-to recipes that you can make in large portions and repurpose for leftovers or meals on the go. If you are ready to go deep and explore some unique and absolutely delicious gourmet preparations, we have some great selections for you here! The recipes are organized into categories for easy reference and rhythm building, but keep in mind one of the great things about keto: You can eat anything, any time of day, without being beholden to regular, grain-based, high-carbohydrate meals as your main source of energy.

You'll learn how to integrate keto staples like bone broth, cauliflower rice, nut milk, and my notorious Bigass Salad into your routine. On the breakfast front, you'll do more than you ever thought possible with eggs (Blueberries and Cream Eggs, anyone?), and learn to make keto-approved substitutes for pancakes, crepes, oatmeal, and muffins. The Soups & Salads section and Veggies & Sides section confirm that a healthy approach to keto is centered on colorful, nutrient-dense plants, contrary to some common mischaracterizations of keto. You'll awaken your creativity in the kitchen with entrées like Jerk Chicken Drumsticks with Cooling Yogurt Sauce (page 146), the Ahi Seaweed Rice Bowl (page 152), and Beef Heart with Mushrooms (page 120; don't be scared, try it!). Recipes in the Appetizers & Small Bites section will make you the most popular person at parties, and are guaranteed to kick-start a conversation about the keto diet. The Lemon Protein Balls (page 218) and Kombucha Gummies (page 217) should pass the picky-kid test with flying colors! You'll whip up some keto-friendly dips, dressings, sauces, and condiments that will go great with vegetables, salads, or entrées. The Beverages section goes way beyond the oft-criticized practice of dumping butter into your coffee to help you create some delicious, nutritious high-fat beverages, including Creamy Keto Hot Chocolate (page 248) and Pumpkin Spice Latte (page 244; sorry Starbucks, we're moving in on you!).

And while I like to say that dessert doesn't need to be a daily routine—especially after a fabulous entrée—habituating yourself away from sugary treats and toward savory preparations can be central to your keto success. Start with the Dairy-Free Avocado Mousse (page 232) or the Coconut-Almond Bites (page 227)! Try new stuff, pick and choose what you like, and tab your favorite pages. Check out 100 more recipes in the back of *The Keto Reset Diet*, and if you have an Instant Pot, be sure to add *The Keto Reset Instant Pot Cookbook* to your collection.

PART 1
GOING KETO

KETO 101

HOW AND WHY KETO WORKS

While "keto" has emerged as the hottest current dietary trend (it recently replaced "paleo" as the most popular diet-related search term on Google), the foundational principles come from the 2.5-million-year scientific study known as human evolution. Evolving the ability to make ketones when calories and carbs were scarce enabled humans to survive through the life-or-death selection pressures they faced in primal times. Go ahead and call it a fad today, but the underpinnings for keto are hardwired into our *Homo sapiens* genes.

When you are fasting or carefully restricting daily carbohydrate intake to under 50 grams per day for a sustained period of time, your liver manufactures a clean-burning alternative energy source called *ketones*. Ketones are metabolized in the body just like glucose, fueling your brain, muscles, and other organs and tissues with an exceptionally clean burning fuel. They also deliver an assortment of additional health benefits. Ketones have a potent anti-inflammatory effect, help suppress the growth of cancerous tumors, improve neurotransmitter and neuron-firing functions in the brain, stimulate the growth of new mitochondria in cells throughout the body, boost internal antioxidant production, and help preserve lean muscle mass from being broken down after strenuous workouts or during periods of fasting. These benefits are so profound that researchers describe ketones as having a signaling effect on your genes, influencing cellular function in a manner similar to, and as powerful as, prescription drugs.

While the remarkable benefits of fasting have been known for decades, it's not a realistic strategy to live in a state of long-term calorie restriction bordering on starvation in order to prompt ketone burning. By adhering to a low-carbohydrate ketogenic eating plan, you can enjoy the longevity benefits of fasting and calorie restriction without having to suffer or starve. Keto helps stabilize hunger and satiety hormones such that adhering to its strict macronutrient guidelines and carb restriction is really and truly no trouble. Optimizing the hormones that regulate appetite, satiety, and fat burning frees the weight loss enthusiast from having to rely on the temporary solution of willpower to restrict calories, for this is a strategy that is destined to fail over the long term.

Eating keto-aligned meals minimizes insulin production and affords the fasting-like benefits of reduced inflammation and more efficient cellular repair and immune function. When you are fasting or keto, you upregulate *autophagy*, the natural cellular detoxification process, as well as *apoptosis*, the (desirable) programmed death of dysfunctional precancerous cells. In contrast, when you rely upon regularly timed, high-carbohydrate meals as your main source of energy for years and decades, your ability to burn fat becomes severely compromised. You exist in a perpetual carbohydrate-dependent, fat-storing mode instead of the efficient fat-burning mode that is our evolutionary genetic preference. In today's default state of carbohydrate dependency, every moderate-to-high-carb snack or meal you consume is met with a surge of insulin into your bloodstream. Any carbs you don't burn immediately are converted in the liver into triglycerides and are then transported by insulin—the body's primary storage hormone—into your fat cells.

Chronically elevated insulin levels (known as *hyperinsulinemia*) render the abundant energy stored in your fat cells inaccessible. Instead, when you burn through the carbs you consumed at breakfast, you get hungry for a snack or a high-carbohydrate lunch. You exist on an energy roller coaster: high-carbohydrate meals for quick energy (usually as soon as you wake up, which locks you into roller-coaster mode all day); the consequent release of insulin, which results in the familiar "sugar crash" as energy is removed from the bloodstream and transported into storage; and the consequent spiking of hunger hormones and fight or flight stress hormones, as your primal genes perceive this drop in blood glucose as a matter of life or death. This hunger spike results in a repeat of the cycle; you crave quick energy carbohydrates in particular to get an energy boost.

Riding the roller coaster every day—instead of becoming an efficient fat burner through dietary modification and supportive exercise, sleep, and stress management habits—leads to the familiar modern affliction known as *burnout*. Perhaps you occasionally, or commonly, experience the afternoon blues at your desk, with a foggy brain and sluggish body? Perhaps you collapse on the couch after a stressful day to engage in hours of passive video entertainment, eating way more popcorn than you thought possible? Perhaps you start conking out after forty minutes of your planned hour-long workout, noticing the telltale sensations of low blood-glucose levels severely compromising your performance? If life sucks when you skip or delay a single meal, this is a sure sign that you are stuck in carbohydrate dependency.

The daily symptoms of carb dependency are no fun, but inside your body, much worse things are happening. Medical experts are in agreement that the catchall disease condition of *metabolic syndrome* is the number-one public health problem of modern times, and that hyperinsulinemia caused by a high-carb diet is the defining characteristic of metabolic syndrome. An estimated 47 million Americans have blood markers indicating metabolic syndrome, which promotes obesity, type 2 diabetes, heart disease, and cancer, and costs over $100 billion annually to treat in the US.

Being stuck in carbohydrate dependency also causes an overstimulation of growth factors in the bloodstream and accelerated cell division. Your body doesn't need to be thrifty or operate with starvation-like efficiency when more energy is constantly coming down the pipe. Since cells divide a given number of times and then die, accelerated cell division and an overstimulation of growth factors such as IGF-1

(insulin-like growth factor) and mTOR (mammalian target of rapamycin) represents the essence of accelerated aging and increased cancer risk.

There is great recognition and agreement among health experts that we are headed for a disaster of epidemic diet-related disease in the years ahead if we don't take drastic steps to escape carbohydrate dependency and improve our ability to burn fat as our primary fuel source—fat obtained from both storage areas on the body and from natural, nutritious dietary fats.

These dietary sources include:

- sustainably raised meat, fish, fowl, and eggs
- high-fat fruits such as avocado, olive, and coconut, and their derivative oils
- the fats contained in nuts, seeds, and their derivative butters
- certain approved modern foods such as high-fat dairy products (butter, cream cheese, raw whole milk, full-fat yogurt, etc.) and dark chocolate with a high cacao percentage

The recipes in this book incorporate all of these healthy ingredients in an amazing array of possibilities such that you will never get bored just because a ketogenic diet limits carb intake. In fact, when you push away the nutrient-deficient sugar and grain filler calories that claim such a large portion of the Standard American Diet (SAD), you open yourself up to a new world of culinary excellence and enjoyment, and access a higher state of general everyday health and disease protection than you ever thought possible. With keto, you can successfully override genetic predispositions toward obesity, type 2 diabetes, and heart disease, an assertion that has been validated in hundreds of respected studies and hundreds of thousands of keto success stories. Visit MarksDailyApple.com to see hundreds of personal stories and stunning before/after photos, like that of Primal Health Coach Tom Misek, who went from 403 pounds to 174, dropping the last 100 pounds with a focused strategy detailed in *The Keto Reset Diet*.

You'll get the best results with this cookbook if you're familiar with *The Keto Reset Diet*. If you don't have the time or inclination to read it, and just can't wait to get into the kitchen and start preparing some "wow" creations, don't worry. We'll give you a quick overview so you can have a basic understanding of how these delicious recipes support the broader health, cognitive function, disease protection, peak athletic performance, and longevity goals of the ketogenic diet, and how you can use keto as the most powerful and effective weight-loss eating strategy ever discovered.

THE LIFELONG BENEFITS OF METABOLIC FLEXIBILITY

By ditching nutrient-deficient, health-destructive, high-insulin-stimulating foods, you start progressing away from carbohydrate dependency and toward fat- and keto-adaptation. As you build momentum over time (the 21-Day Metabolism Reset detailed in *The Keto Reset Diet* will help you make great progress in a short time!), you will develop what I call *metabolic flexibility*—the ability to burn a variety of fuel sources to meet your body's needs at any given time—regardless of whether or not you eat regular meals.

The metabolic flexibility that you establish during the Metabolism Reset can be fine-tuned by intermittent fasting, where you turbocharge fat burning (and eventually ketone burning) and force your body to burn internal sources of energy. There are no strict rules for fasting—you can skip breakfast on certain days of the week or randomly skip meals so you subsist comfortably on one or two meals a day instead of three. For example, I fast every time I travel, because it helps me beat jet lag and because the food available in airports doesn't appeal to me. I also generally operate in a compressed eating window wherein I skip breakfast every day (okay, I have coffee with cream and a pinch of sugar in the morning, along with my *Miami Herald* crossword puzzle), and consume my calories between 1 p.m. and 7 p.m.

Whatever pattern you choose, keep in mind that you first have to reset your metabolism to prefer fat before you engage in purposeful fasting for metabolic flexibility. Fasting while still carbohydrate dependent will simply activate the fight or flight response, and you will break down lean muscle tissue and convert it into glucose to fuel your energy needs, via a process known as *gluconeogenesis*. This leads to the familiar destination known as burnout, as mentioned previously.

Once you have obtained an impressive level of metabolic flexibility, as evidenced by your ability to skip meals and feel great, you can commence a formal period of nutritional ketosis lasting a minimum of six weeks. Here, you will target protein intake (averaging 0.7 grams per pound of lean body mass per day for most people—that is, about 70 to 85 grams of protein per day to start, although some people might need more or less depending on their size and physical activity), limit carbohydrate intake to 50 grams per day or below, and eat enough nutritious fats to feel satisfied at all times.

Keto pioneer Luis Villasenor of Ketogains.com (who has been bodybuilding and powerlifting for sixteen years and counting while adhering to a ketogenic diet!) says that a proper approach to keto entails making protein a "target," carbohydrate a "limit," and fat a "lever" to enable total dietary satisfaction at all times. That means you make sure to eat enough protein, not too many carbs, and however much fat you need to achieve your health, weight loss, and fitness goals. While keto definitely requires a delicate, precise (okay, let's say "strict"!) approach, and is ill-advised for anyone who is not fully prepared, it is never, ever about struggling, suffering, or exercising massive willpower to get through the day. When you minimize insulin and upregulate fat burning, *you will hardly ever feel hungry*, and when you do it will be a manageable recognition that it is time to eat, not an all-consuming (no pun intended) desire to slam some food before you snap. This is why keto is so easy to adhere to when you do it correctly, and why it is so effective for fat reduction.

When you complete this Keto Reset journey as described, you will have attained a level of metabolic flexibility that will benefit you the rest of your life, even if in the future you choose to consume more carbs than keto guidelines specify. Your body desperately wants to burn fat, and fights valiantly to preserve health under the wildly excessive carb-intake patterns that are typical of modern diets, but that are a serious affront to our genetic expectations. Once you get good at fat burning, you will preserve this skill to a large extent for a long time—like typing or riding a bike. This is perhaps the greatest beauty of keto: You can call upon it any time as a tool to hone metabolic flexibility, recalibrate if you happen to go through a period of indulgence, drop some excess body fat that crept back into the picture, correct disease risk factors in your blood results, achieve targeted benefits for athletic performance and recovery, and generally promote longevity in a manner more profound than virtually anything else known to science.

LOSING EXCESS BODY FAT WITH KETO

Becoming fat- and keto-adapted is the only true way to lose excess body fat, keep it off long-term, and not ever stress about this most frustrating issue again. Unfortunately, the traditional "calories in/calories out" approach of combining obsessive and regimented calorie restriction with exhaustive exercise has proven over the last several decades to be a dismal failure.

When you deprive a carbohydrate-dependent body of its usual primary fuel source, you trigger a prolonged activation of the fight or flight response, which in turn triggers gluconeogenesis (the breakdown of lean muscle into glucose instead of the more desirable shift to ketones when you become fat- and keto-adapted). With a low-carb crash diet, you'll lose weight initially from reduced cellular inflammation and water retention, glycogen depletion, diminished lean muscle mass, and even burning some stored body fat, but you are headed for disaster when your exhausted, depleted, still-carbohydrate-dependent body tries to recover from this episode of extreme metabolic stress/starvation by overeating and being less active and more sleepy in daily life.

This is the sad story that even the most devoted and health-conscious dieter has likely experienced many times over. The more it happens, the more metabolic damage you incur, such that you program your genes to become expert at holding on to your precious fat stores instead of burning them—even when you try to control portions and exercise with devotion! Furthermore, even an exhausting fitness regimen typically has little or no impact on your fat-reduction goals. While there are numerous health benefits to be gained by being fit, efficient reduction of excess body fat is not one of them. Vigorous workouts have been shown to stimulate a corresponding increase in appetite and also prompt you to become generally less active and more lazy throughout the day.

These surprising dynamics play out both consciously and subconsciously over the course of the day. For example, you may make the conscious decision to reward yourself after a tough gym session by dropping by the coffee shop, where your venti frappuccino can deliver hundreds more calories than you burned at spin class and double the carbs of keto's daily limit! Subconsciously, you might experience an annoying recurring pattern of a predawn, high-energy group workout paired with an evening glued to the couch, finishing off a pint of ice cream instead of just a quick episode and a quick scoop. This stuff is not mere conjecture, but rather a scientifically validated phenomenon known as the *compensation theory of exercise*.

When you pursue metabolic flexibility and distinct periods of nutritional ketosis, you are going to attack the cause of excess body fat, rather than fussing over the symptom of storing more calories than you eat. What your keto lifestyle will enable is *hormone optimization*—a stabilization of appetite, energy levels, cognition, and mood all day long, regardless of whether you eat regular meals. Indeed, fasting, skipping meals, eating in a spontaneous, intuitive manner rather than a regimented manner, and indulging occasionally and then getting right back on track the next day (or the next week, if you're like me and enjoy a total cultural immersion while on vacation) are what I believe to be the fundamental benefits of keto.

BACON AND BUTTER? NOT SO FAST!

Unfortunately, in the aggressive promotion and hype surrounding keto, the fasting component of a ketogenic lifestyle is often overlooked. Instead, misguided promoters and enthusiasts seem to be equating keto with stuffing one's face with high-fat foods and beverages. No wonder detractors disparage keto as the bacon and butter diet! To clarify, ketones are produced in the liver under the unique and fragile circumstances of having low levels of insulin, blood sugar, and liver glycogen. The best way to get into ketosis is to fast, because you are restricting both carbohydrates and total energy. This prompts you to accelerate internal energy production mechanisms such as mobilization of free fatty acids from storage depots into the bloodstream, and the manufacture of ketones in the liver. Of course, you don't want to starve in the name of keto, so consuming ample dietary fats as your primary energy source helps you enjoy the long scientifically validated benefits of fasting (improved cellular repair, enhanced immune function, accelerated fat burning, and reduced inflammation) without having to starve yourself.

If you go hog wild (literally, with the hall pass on bacon consumption) and overconsume high-fat meals, beverages, and snacks, you won't lose excess body fat, because your body has plenty of energy from dietary calories. Hence, the optimal approach to losing excess body fat with keto is to first patiently build your metabolic flexibility via the Keto Reset journey, without struggling, suffering, or backsliding. Only then can you contemplate a purposeful caloric deficit to shed excess pounds. The caloric deficit is always from dietary fat, because carbs are already limited to under 50 grams and protein is always targeted at 0.7 grams per pound of lean body mass to meet your basic needs for metabolic function. With some mindfulness at meals and adherence to fasting in the morning until you experience true sensations of hunger, you'll be able to attain your ideal body composition and maintain it for years to come.

HOW TO DO KETO THE RIGHT WAY AND AVOID BACKSLIDES AND BURNOUT

The wonderful lifelong benefits of keto are available to all of us, as we humans are genetically hardwired to cope with prolonged periods of caloric and/or carbohydrate restriction. However, a lifetime of carbohydrate-dependent eating patterns has to be unwound carefully—that's why I present the multistep Keto Reset approach, where you must demonstrate a requisite level of metabolic fitness before proceeding along successive steps to an eventual extended foray into nutritional ketosis. Unfortunately, the instant gratification mind-set in modern culture often leads to an overly stressful, sink or swim approach to dietary transformation that is doomed to fail.

Fortunately, going keto is easier and less arduous than it sounds. Yes, you are going to say goodbye to many of your high-carb comfort foods and bring a greater level of awareness to your food choices at all times to stay in keto. However, you are almost never going to feel hungry (and especially not "hangry"—clever jargon of the low-carb community to convey that a bad mood goes hand in hand with hunger swings); you will enjoy delicious, diverse, and highly satisfying meals; and you will experience authentic fat reduction, which will keep you focused and motivated to stay on track.

If you find yourself struggling with energy lulls or carbohydrate cravings, you can usually make quick fixes to boost your progress. For example, increasing your intake of sodium, potassium, and magnesium to adjust for a reduction in inflammation and water retention in cells throughout the body can help break you out of recurring fatigue patterns.

The Keto Reset takes a gradual approach because I hope this will become a lifestyle change rather than just another quick-fix diet. If you require a little more patience in the 21-Day Metabolism Reset mode (described in more detail in a later section) so that it becomes a 42-Day Reset, so be it. Once you realize the benefits of becoming fat- and keto-adapted, you'll see why it is worth taking the time to do correctly.

LIVING A KETO-FRIENDLY LIFESTYLE

As I advocate for patience in your approach to keto, I also encourage you to relax and reject the obsessive, overly stressful approach that seems to be quite common with dietary transformation programs these days. While it's important to have an accurate feel for the relative carbohydrate and protein content of your favorite meals and snacks, I strongly advise against a regimented approach that can easily become too stressful and frustrating. I'd rather discuss a more relaxed big-picture objective of living a keto-friendly lifestyle. This entails exercising sensibly, prioritizing sleep above everything else, and implementing effective stress management techniques. If you instead exercise in chronic patterns, have less than optimal sleeping habits, and get stressed and harried

easily, these behaviors will push you back in the direction of carbohydrate dependency, even if you make devoted efforts to transform your diet.

When your lifestyle behaviors are optimized, and you have successfully completed the Keto Reset so you are comfortably fat- and keto-adapted, you can implement a dietary strategy that I like to call eating in the "keto zone," which is less daunting than making a precise effort to maintain nutritional ketosis indefinitely. Being in the keto zone entails a general pattern of eating wholesome, nutrient-dense foods (yes, even carbs!); eliminating nutrient-deficient refined grains, sugars, and oils; getting comfortable with intermittent fasting—whether spontaneous or scheduled; and not obsessing about measuring blood ketones or monitoring every single gram of carbohydrates you consume. When you eat in the keto zone, your daily carbohydrate intake might range from under 50 grams per day when you are fasting or making a focused effort to sustain nutritional ketosis, to up near 150 grams when you are not in a distinct keto phase and are more liberal with your carbohydrate consumption. For example, opting for some sweet potato fries with your steak dinner, enjoying heaps of fresh berries from the farmers' market during the summer, or even finding your way to some freshly made gelato during a European vacation.

As I mention in detail in my Primal Blueprint books and online educational courses, if you simply ditch grains and sugars, it's pretty difficult to exceed the primal-approved upper limit of 150 grams of carbs on average per day during non-keto phases. This affords abundant consumption of vegetables as well as healthy amounts of nutrient-dense carbs like fresh seasonal fruit, sweet potatoes, quinoa, and wild rice, along with the incidental carbs found in nuts and seeds and their derivative butters, high-cacao-percentage dark chocolate, coconut milk, other nutritious foods, and even occasional treats. Even when you are hard-core keto and staying under 50 grams of carbs per day, you can still consume abundant servings of assorted above-ground vegetables (such as leafy greens and those in the cruciferous family) and a reasonable amount of incidental carbs, and still land safely under 50 grams.

This relaxed keto zone approach arises from extensive experimentation by me as well as members of my team, and from the feedback of thousands of enthusiasts on our Keto Reset Facebook group. There is certainly nothing bad about maintaining a state of nutritional ketosis long-term; doing so may be of most benefit to those with a history of metabolic damage and/or difficulty reducing excess body fat, those trying to manage disease conditions like cancer or epilepsy, or those with distinct endurance performance goals who want to become less dependent on glucose during sustained exercise.

There is plenty of debate and controversy surrounding assertions such as these, so I encourage you to self-experiment and determine what makes you look, feel, and perform your best, and to never allow anxiety or negativity to enter the picture when it comes to eating. Eating your personal favorites from the list of foods that are optimal for human health should always be considered one of the great pleasures of life. If your meals deliver anything less than total pleasure and satisfaction, your approach is flawed and destined for failure at some time in the future, full stop. Relax, enjoy life, pay attention to how good foods make you feel good, and how junk foods make you feel lousy after those few moments of pleasure when they hit your taste buds. Bring more mindfulness to your eating habits as you focus on pleasure and enjoyment rather than making your meals akin to refueling stops at the gas station. I'm confident that your best results will come when you strictly eliminate the inflammatory, nutrient-deficient, insulin-stimulating, fatigue-generating grains, sugars, and refined high polyunsaturated vegetable oils, and emphasize the nutrient-dense foods humans were designed to eat, such as colorful plants and natural, nutritious fats.

THE 21-DAY METABOLISM RESET— THE JOURNEY TO KETO

R eady to take action? Here we go on the Keto Reset journey! Following is an overview of the 21-Day Metabolism Reset, the fine-tuning period and midterm exam, and a six-week nutritional ketosis period.

STAGE 1: THE 21-DAY METABOLISM RESET

The first three weeks of your journey help you ditch dietary and lifestyle practices that keep you dependent on carbohydrates, and instead progress toward fat-adaptation. No matter who you are or what your starting point, you can make a remarkable amount of progress in only three weeks, but it's going to take some sincere focus and dedication to depart from eating habits that have become ingrained (pun intended) over decades. It's also going to take much more than honoring the basic dos and don'ts with your food choices. Your exercise, sleep, and stress management practices will make or break your success with dietary transformation.

As detailed in *The Keto Reset Diet,* the most basic and health-critical initial step in the journey toward optimum health, vitality, disease protection, and longevity is to ditch grains, sugars, and refined high polyunsaturated vegetable oils—the "big three" worst offenders in the modern diet. I urge you to make a sincere commitment to a total elimination of these offensive agents out of the gate so that you can move your body out of a carbohydrate-dependency state and recalibrate to make fat and ketones your preferred fuel source. In particular, a half-hearted attempt to ditch grains and sugars brings a high risk of backsliding because of the addictive properties of both sugar (described in *The Case Against Sugar* by Gary Taubes and *Fat Chance* by Dr. Robert Lustig) and wheat (described in the books *Wheat Belly* by Dr. William Davis and *Grain Brain* by Dr. David Perlmutter). Remember, the body burns glucose quickly and easily, thrusting you onto a roller coaster that's difficult to dismount.

Over the long term, strive to strictly limit sweets and treats, recognizing that a few moments of gustatory pleasure often results in many hours of unpleasant physical symptoms, not to mention the psychological distress of behaving in a manner incongruent with your stated goals. If you do happen to indulge occasionally, strive to enjoy smaller portions with full attention and appreciation, instead of mindless chowing. When it comes to grains, use them incidentally instead of as meal centerpieces—particularly if you have symptoms of gluten sensitivity or leaky gut syndrome. Look for recipes in this book and others that have creative and delicious alternatives to grain-based comfort foods. For example, using pan-fried sliced vegetables in place of pasta noodles, or finely chopped cauliflower in place of rice.

It's urgent to eliminate all forms of refined vegetable and seed oils, and the processed foods that contain them. Bottled forms include canola, soybean, corn, sunflower, and safflower oils, and you can find these sinister agents on the labels of many processed, packaged, and frozen foods. While completely eliminating oils might be impossible due to hidden sources and their common use in restaurants, you can certainly strive for zero tolerance at home and high vigilance outside the home. After all, vegetable oils provide no flavor satisfaction and cause an immediate disturbance in healthy cardiovascular function on a level similar to smoking a cigarette, according to *Deep Nutrition* author Dr. Cate Shanahan. While cultural forces and manipulative marketing are against you in this effort to eat cleanly (some resources still tout canola as healthy despite compelling evidence to the contrary), take inspiration from many keto enthusiasts who never eat these foods, and know that you will find none of those offensive ingredients anywhere in this book.

Yes, it's time to literally grab a garbage can and start tossing things out of your pantry and refrigerator. Of particular importance to eliminate are sweetened beverages of all kinds, because they stimulate a big insulin response without making you feel full like a solid food would. Sodas are obviously out of the picture, but so are the sports drinks, energy drinks, fruit juices, and designer coffees that we don't normally equate with soda in the sugar bomb category. Examine labels and notice the massive carbohydrate content of sweetened drinks. Even certain types of kombucha have so much added sugar that they are similar to a Vitamin Water. And a Vitamin Water is similar in fructose content to a Coke! Choose water, coffee, herbal tea, or unsweetened kombucha for your beverages.

You'll also dutifully get rid of all grains and foods made with grains, including wheat, rice, corn, pasta, and cereal. Sugars and all the processed, packaged, and frozen snacks and treats made with added sugar are also out. You cannot allow even the smallest leakage during this 21-Day Metabolism Reset, or you will drift back in the direction of carbohydrate dependency. Remember, consuming high-carbohydrate meals stimulates insulin, which hinders fat metabolism. Once you burn through the carbohydrates from your meal, you will start to crave more because with all that insulin in your bloodstream, the stored energy in your fat cells is inaccessible.

Once you complete your purge, you will have the enjoyable experience of immediately restocking with colorful, nutrient-dense, primal-approved foods, focusing on meat, fish, poultry, and eggs; vegetables and a moderate amount of in-season fruit (dark berries preferred); nuts, avocados, coconuts, and derivative butters and oils; high-fat dairy if tolerated; perhaps small amounts of quinoa and wild rice; and 85% cacao or higher dark chocolate. Opt for the highest quality ingredients you can afford (grass-fed and pastured meat and eggs; organic or pesticide-free produce; bean-to-bar, fair-trade chocolate; and so on). While keto is another level of sophistication beyond primal/paleo, we don't even worry about devoted carb restriction out of the gate. Instead, we focus on replacing unhealthy carb sources with a sufficient level of nutrient-dense carbs to make your transition painless.

During week two, you will turn your attention to the complementary lifestyle factors that can make or break your success with keto: exercise, sleep, and stress management. Following are some highlights to get each of these three objectives dialed in:

EXERCISE: The major objectives here are to increase all forms of general everyday movement, which helps turbocharge fat metabolism, and avoid anything resembling an overly stressful chronic exercise pattern, which pushes you strongly back toward carbohydrate dependency. Walking around more, going back and forth from a sitting desk position to a standup desk, doing flexibility/mobility exercises (stretching, yoga, Pilates, calisthenics), and conducting comfortably paced cardiovascular exercises help you prioritize fat as your primary fuel choice, because your body burns mostly fat during low-intensity exercise. For cardio enthusiasts, the cutoff point between a comfortable fat-burning session and a more stressful glucose-burning session is a heart rate of *180* minus *your age* = beats per minute. For example, a forty-year-old exerciser would observe an upper limit of 140 beats per minute (180 minus 40) in order to qualify as a minimally stressful, predominantly fat-burning session. This fat-burning maximum heart rate is surprisingly moderate and easy to achieve even during a brisk walk for most people, or a casual jog for accomplished runners. Yes, slowing down really does help you lose excess body fat!

In contrast, cardio enthusiasts who exercise often at medium-to-difficult intensity, such as with group exercise classes, or jogging or cycling group outings, get really competent at burning glucose because a greater percentage of glucose is burned as you escalate exercise intensity. Depleting, glucose-burning workouts leave you craving sugar in the hours afterward, seriously compromising your keto goals. In fact, it's also recommended that you tone down the overall energy expenditure of your workouts when you are involved in a dietary transformation. When you first go keto, your muscles and brain compete for precious ketone energy, since their usual supply of glucose has been cut off. When you become fully fat- and keto-adapted over time, your muscles transition to burning mostly fatty acids, prioritizing ketones for use by the brain (because the brain can't burn fat, only glucose or the glucose replacement of ketones).

SLEEP: The most urgent objective with sleep is to minimize your exposure to artificial light and digital stimulation after dark, the combination of which is a disastrous affront to our hardwired genetic expectation to align sleep and wake cycles with the rising and setting of the sun. Creating a mellow, dark, relaxing evening routine will help recalibrate your hormones to become more aligned with your natural circadian rhythm, which entails waking up around sunrise full of energy, and slowing down and eventually getting sleepy soon after it gets dark—as our ancestors did for a couple million years. This is important not just to ensure optimal sleep, but also to transition out of the all-too-common evening sugar cravings and fat-storage hormonal patterns.

STRESS MANAGEMENT: Surprising as it may seem, operating at a hectic pace, multitasking, hyperconnecting, or having difficult personal interactions actually compromise your ability to burn fat, because they stimulate the fight or flight response that goes hand in hand with sugar burning. In *The Keto Reset Diet*, an assortment of suggestions are offered to help you balance your hectic pace with necessary downtime. Realize that even vigorous workouts that are often touted as a "stress release" are merely another form of stress to your body. It's essential to carve out time in your schedule for true rest and relaxation: walking the dog around the block each evening, doing a few minutes of morning meditation, sitting on a park bench and watching the birds for ten minutes at lunchtime, or conducting some deep-breathing exercises at your desk after intense phone calls, meetings, or periods of sustained cognitive focus.

Beyond the inclusion of breaks into your daily routine, you'll be inspired to nurture meaningful face-to-face social connections, de-emphasizing excessive use of technology and social media in the process. You'll learn how to use technology to make your life easier and less stressful instead of falling victim to the destructive effects of being hyperconnected. You'll find more ways to have fun and keep your motivations pure with your lifestyle transformation goals. Consider keeping a gratitude journal, and carve out time for just *you*—enjoying hobbies or simply decompressing with some precious moments in nature.

Since the objectives of the first two weeks are very ambitious and all encompassing, week three of the Reset will be all about catching your breath and settling into a routine whereby you enjoy and appreciate your food choices, workout patterns, sleeping routines, and stress-management practices. This is a chance to take a closer look at any lingering need-to-improve areas, whether it's been blasting your eyeballs with screen light late in the evening or still adding a couple/few/several pumps of peach sweetener to your iced tea. If you are inexperienced in any areas of the Reset, you will take some time to quantify things like your exercise heart rate or the macronutrient composition of your meals. Nothing too strict or daunting, just building your skills so you have a feel for what a proper aerobic workout feels like or what a day of 150 grams of carbs or 0.7 grams of protein per pound of lean body mass looks like.

STAGE 2: FINE-TUNING PERIOD AND MIDTERM EXAM

After completing a successful 21-Day Reset, you should have some reliable indicators that you are escaping the sinister influence of carbohydrate dependency and progressing toward fat-adaptation: lower body weight due to increased fat metabolism and a reduction in inflammation and water retention; an ability to comfortably delay your morning meal for a few hours or more; more stable energy, mood, cognition, and appetite throughout the day; diminished cravings for quick-energy carbohydrates; and perhaps improvements in digestive or autoimmune conditions.

During this fine-tuning period, you will enhance your metabolic flexibility by delaying your morning meal for as long as comfortably possible, ideally making it until midday with stable energy and peak cognitive function without having to eat, at least on some days. Again, this is not a contest to merely survive until noon, weak and famished and staring at the clock until you can gorge. Instead, you are simply tracking your level of metabolic flexibility by noticing how long you can last until you experience true sensations of hunger.

In *The Keto Reset Diet*, a midterm exam is presented where you are asked to answer a series of subjective questions relating to your level of metabolic flexibility. You give yourself a score of 1 to 10 for your level of alignment with questions like "Have you eliminated grains and sugars from your diet?," and "Can you fast comfortably from 8 p.m. to 12 p.m. the following day?" If you score 75 percent or better, this is an excellent indication that you are ready to handle the rigors of more devoted carb restriction and nutritional ketosis.

STAGE 3: NUTRITIONAL KETOSIS PERIOD

Going keto is the exciting final step in the journey toward building the highest level of metabolic flexibility and maintaining this attribute for years to come. Here, the objective is to carefully limit carb intake to 50 grams per day or below, target protein intake at 0.7 grams per pound of lean body mass, and eat sufficient amounts of nutritious natural fats to feel satisfied at every meal. Keto should never be a struggle to fight through hunger, intense cravings, or recurring fatigue. However, the level of focus and commitment will be much higher than a normal pattern of primal-aligned eating.

Ketosis is a sensitive metabolic state that can be disrupted for a prolonged period of time by even a moderate ingestion of carbs. Some studies from Drs. Phinney and Volek, pioneers in the study of how low-carbohydrate diets benefit athletes, suggest that it takes many novice keto enthusiasts up to a week to return to ketosis after a carbohydrate departure. Seasoned veterans of keto report that they can return to a state of ketosis after a prolonged overnight fast and a couple of keto-aligned meals. They are referencing readings from portable blood ketone meters where subjects exceed the minimum keto threshold of 0.5 mmol/L.

A minimum six-week commitment is requested because this is the duration necessary to obtain maximum benefits and also to gain the proper momentum so keto is easy and enjoyable to maintain. Unfortunately, many people struggle and bail out after about three weeks of keto. With the initial euphoria and enthusiasm carrying you through the early days, you may have a bit of an energy dip at three weeks, since it's no small feat to reprogram your genes to burn fat instead of indulging their lifelong preference for carbs. As you continue forward with your adherence to ketogenic eating patterns, your fat- and ketone-burning systems upregulate and things get easier and easier. If you can have the faith and resilience to stay focused when you hit the three-week mark, you will create some real momentum over the next three weeks.

At the six-week mark, you will have achieved an elite level of metabolic flexibility—congratulations! You have successfully reprogrammed your genes to prefer fat for fuel (either from storage when you fast, or from the natural, nutritious dietary fats) and are expert at manufacturing whatever ketones you need to sustain cognitive function when you are fasting or eating low-carb meals. Some enthusiasts decide to continue in a ketogenic eating pattern indefinitely, while others like to experiment with adding back nutritious carbs and dialing in a preferred intake level. This carb intake level depends on your fitness and body composition goals, overall health, personal genetics, and assorted other lifestyle variables and preferences. As previously discussed, operating in the keto zone is sufficient to sustain optimal metabolic flexibility, effortless long-term maintenance of ideal body composition, and profound benefits in immune function, inflammation control, and cognitive function.

This Keto Reset journey might sound a little involved, but the truth is you will get into a good groove and experience immediate positive feedback when you ditch carbohydrate dependency. Many enthusiasts report that they feel free from emotional stress, negativity, and obsessions with meals and calorie counting when they go keto. For the first time, they are able to tap into internal energy stores, get off the carbohydrate-insulin roller coaster, and enjoy a productive life without worrying about food.

THE DOS
AND DON'TS
OF KETO

This section guides you away from nutrient-deficient, high-carb snacks, condiments, and meal staples and offers suggestions for integrating keto-friendly foods into your game.

DITCHING GRAINS, SUGARS, AND REFINED OILS

The big three offenders are ubiquitous in processed, packaged, and frozen foods; in restaurant and fast-food offerings; and even in "healthy" stuff from natural foods markets. I can't tell you how many times I learn from enthusiasts or friends who claim to be on a strict primal diet that it includes objectionable products like celebrity "red wine and olive oil" salad dressing (made with refined vegetable oil), nondairy creamers made with corn syrup, or healthy organic energy bars with massive doses of carbohydrates.

OILS TO ELIMINATE: Refined high polyunsaturated vegetable and seed oils (canola, corn, soybean, sunflower, safflower, etc.); butter-substitute spreads and sprays (margarine, Smart Balance, Promise); processed and packaged food containing vegetable oils or trans fats (partially hydrogenated fats).

REFINED GRAIN PRODUCTS TO ELIMINATE: Baguettes, cereal, corn, crackers, croissants, danishes, donuts, energy bars, frozen snacks and meals, graham crackers, granola bars, muffins, pasta, pizza, pretzels, protein bars, rice, rolls, saltine crackers, tortillas, Triscuits, Wheat Thins, chips (corn, potato, tortilla), cooking grains (amaranth, barley, bulgur, couscous, millet, rye), puffed snacks (Cheetos, Goldfish, Pirate's Booty, popcorn, rice cakes).

REFINED SUGAR PRODUCTS TO ELIMINATE: Agave syrup, brown sugar, cane sugar, evaporated cane sugar, fruit bars and rolls, high-fructose corn syrup, honey, molasses, powdered sugar, raw sugar.

INTEGRATING KETO-FRIENDLY FOODS

Ketogenic eating is ultralow in carbohydrates, moderate in protein, and high in natural, nutritious fats. Choose the foods you prefer from this ancestral-inspired list of meat, fish, poultry, eggs, vegetables, fruits, nuts and seeds, and assorted approved modern foods such as high-fat dairy products and high-cacao-percentage dark chocolate.

APPROVED FATS

- High-fat fruits such as avocados, coconuts, olives, and their derivative oils
- Nuts, seeds, and their derivative butters and nondairy milks
- Fatty cuts of meat from naturally raised animals
- Fish, especially oily cold water fish from the SMASH hits group (sardines, mackerel, anchovies, salmon, herring)
- Butter, ghee, lard, bacon fat, and tallow

APPROVED CARBOHYDRATES

Generally, you can make high-fiber, above-ground vegetables such as the leafy green and cruciferous family (broccoli, Brussels sprouts, cabbage, kale, etc.) a dietary centerpiece. These foods are some of the most nutrient-dense on the planet and also support a healthy intestinal microbiome. Due to their high fiber and water content, they do not stimulate the insulin response that can compromise keto efforts. While I recommend staying below 50 grams of carbohydrates per day, you can give yourself a free pass to consume as many above-ground, high-fiber vegetables and avocados as you want. In contrast, carbohydrates from foods that are starchier or calorically denser should be limited during formal nutritional ketosis efforts. These include many carbohydrates that offer tremendous nutritional benefits and are an acceptable part of a general primal/paleo-style eating strategy, but will quickly push you over the keto limit—foods like fruit, wild rice, quinoa, and the starchier vegetables like squash, beets, rutabaga, and sweet potato. Keep in mind that because carbohydrates are a *limit*, there is no need to aim for 50 grams per day. When you eat a colorful, varied diet, your carbohydrate intake will naturally vary from day to day. Some days you might eat very few carbohydrates, while other days you might bump up against your 50-gram cap.

KETO-FRIENDLY SNACKS

- Avocado with salt and lime juice
- Basic Bone Broth (page 35)
- Coconut butter: an absolute delicacy, hard to find but super delicious and nutritious. Look for Nikki's brand, since it has numerous exotic flavors.
- Dark chocolate: gradually habituate to 85% or higher cacao. To ensure the highest quality product, look for cacao beans as the first ingredient and/or the "Bean-to-Bar" designation, as well as a "Fair Trade" designation on the box.

- Hard-boiled egg
- Jerky: high-quality beef or other meat, without sweeteners, nitrates, preservatives, or other chemicals
- Nuts, seeds, and their derivative butters
- Oily, cold-water fish: remember SMASH (sardines, mackerel, anchovies, salmon, herring)
- Olives packed in olive oil (avoid canola and sunflower oils)
- Pork rinds/chicharrones: natural ingredients only, no chemicals, bad oils, or sweeteners
- Primal Kitchen keto bars (PrimalKitchen.com)
- Trail mix: Use raw or dry-roasted nuts, seeds, unsweetened coconut flakes, 85% cacao dark chocolate pieces or cacao nibs, small amounts of unsweetened dried fruit, and a dash of Himalayan sea salt
- Vegetables dipped in guacamole or natural almond or peanut butter

RECIPE REPLACEMENT IDEAS

Some of the recipes in this book are designed to simulate your favorite grain-based recipes with keto-approved replacement ingredients. Many keto enthusiasts assert that the grain replacements taste better than the original grain-based preparations! Here are some swap-outs at a glance (you'll see more as you dig into the recipes):

GRAIN REPLACEMENTS

- Coconut flour or almond meal for wheat flour
- Lettuce or collard leaves for tortillas or buns
- Spiralized veggies for pasta

SWEETENER REPLACEMENTS

- Citrus (lemon, lime or orange) zest or juice
- Dark cocoa powder
- Spices—cinnamon, vanilla extract, ginger, salt, pepper
- Nut and seed butters
- Stevia, erythritol, or monkfruit for chemically altered sweeteners or sugary sweeteners
- Unsweetened shredded (or flaked) coconut

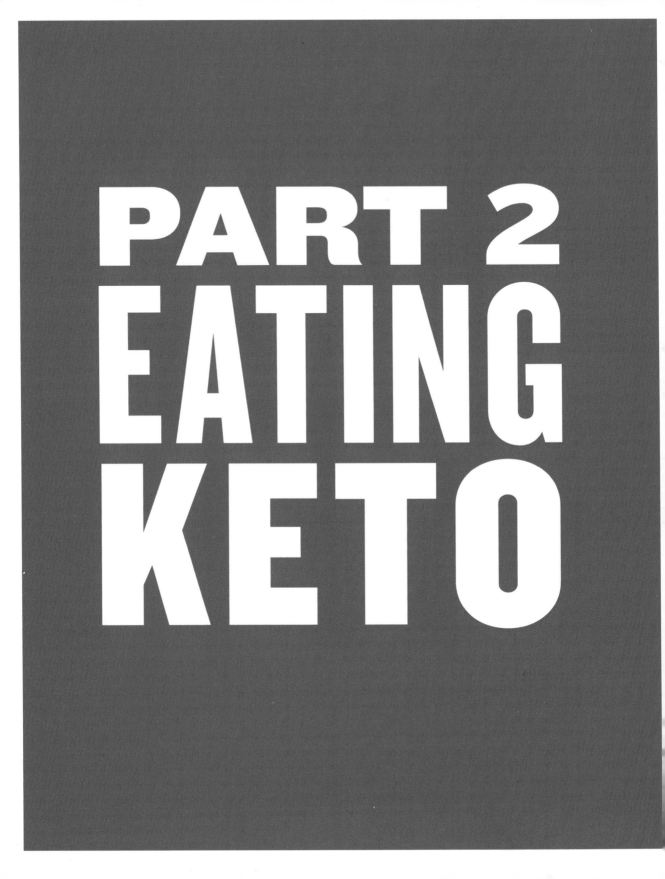

KETO RESET STAPLES

TIP: Keep a large zippered plastic bag in your freezer, and whenever you have vegetable scraps such as the leaves and bottoms of celery, leaves and ends of carrots, broccoli stems, and so on, toss them in the bag. You can do the same with leftover bones and skin. This way you always have ingredients on hand when you want to make a batch of bone broth.

3. To rapidly cool the broth, fill your kitchen sink with ice water. Place a metal bowl in the ice water and place a metal sieve or colander over the bowl. Carefully strain the hot broth into the bowl (discard the solids). Allow it to chill for about 15 minutes, stirring occasionally.

4. Optional: Strain the broth again through a fine-mesh sieve into a spouted measuring cup. Pour the broth into mason jars, leaving about 1 inch of headspace. Secure the lids and place the jars immediately in the refrigerator or freezer. (Alternatively, you can pour the broth into ice cube trays or silicone molds and freeze it.) Use refrigerated broth within a few days.

KETO RESET STAPLES

BONE BROTH

We're hot for bone broth in the primal and keto communities! Bone broth is one of the most nutrient-dense foods on the planet, packed with vitamins, minerals, prebiotic fiber, and special compounds like collagen and glycosaminoglycans that nurture joints and connective tissue in the body. The latter are extremely difficult to obtain from other dietary sources, even for hard-core meat eaters. Unfortunately, the Standard American Diet (SAD) has completely disregarded bone broth and organ meats in favor of consuming mainly the leanest possible cuts of meat. This conventional-wisdom recommendation to avoid the most nutritious parts of animals in favor of a narrow focus on lean flesh is motivated by the idea of avoiding the long-dreaded saturated fat. As the dated and oversimplified "lipid hypothesis of heart disease" goes, consuming saturated fat and cholesterol increases your risk of heart disease, because the plaques that form in arteries contain these agents.

The idea that fat and cholesterol are unhealthy has been almost completely shattered by respected science examining the dietary practices of large populations for decades. The Framingham Heart Study and Nurses' Health Study are prominent examples that reveal no correlation between dietary fat and cholesterol intake and heart disease. In his book, *Why We Get Fat*, Gary Taubes relates emphatically that there has never been a single study ever published to show that consuming saturated fat by itself is unhealthy. As enthusiasts in the ancestral health community know, fat and cholesterol do bad things in the body only when they are consumed in a high-carbohydrate, high insulin producing diet!

Unfortunately, even experts in the paleo community have advocated for choosing lean meats, observing that today's industrialized animals are fatter than the Paleolithic animals our ancestors ate. What's overlooked with this recommendation is that our ancestors routinely extracted every bit of edible nutrition from the animals they consumed—enjoying organ meats that deliver considerably more nutrient density than flesh, and extracting the highly beneficial agents in bone and joint material—as happens when you make bone broth. This "nose to tail" animal consumption results in more fat and vastly more nutritional benefits than opting for chicken breast and ultralean hamburgers in the name of health.

Dr. Cate Shanahan, author of the highly acclaimed *Deep Nutrition*, mentions meat on the bone (which includes bone broth) and organ meats as two of the four essential food categories for an optimal human diet, the other pillars being fresh foods and fermented foods. Clearly, the SAD is woefully inadequate in all four categories, and even many enthusiastic primal/paleo style eaters can fall short in one or more categories. Getting into the bone broth scene can help bring your already healthy eating habits to the next level. Enjoying a warm and deeply satisfying mug of bone broth in the morning might eventually have more appeal than a harried grab of a sugary Starbucks concoction during your morning commute. Since many healthy-living enthusiasts have "discovered" this ancient remedy of bone broth, there are more and more high-quality products popping up on grocery store shelves. However, it's also easy and inexpensive to make your own. All you need is a carcass from last night's turkey or chicken, or a visit to your local butcher or grocery meat department to procure some fun stuff like cow joints, chicken feet, or turkey necks. The joint material is usually super cheap—one meat specialty store I frequent packages cow joints exclusively for their canine customers (or the financially responsible party of the canine customer!). For a few bucks, you can walk out with the best raw material for bone broth.

BASIC BONE BROTH

One of the best ways to enjoy bone broth is simply hot out of a mug. You can also use your broth to make Golden Bone Broth (page 247) or Garlicky Bone Broth (page 246), or the many delicious soups you will find later in this book!

MAKES 8 TO 12 CUPS (DEPENDING ON THE METHOD)

8 to 16 ounces beef or poultry bones, or the carcass from a whole chicken or turkey

2 to 4 tablespoons tomato paste (if making beef broth)

5 to 10 ounces vegetable scraps (see Tip) or 1 large onion (roughly chopped, including skin and root end if organic), 2 stalks celery (roughly chopped, including leaves), and 2 carrots (roughly chopped, including leafy tops)

2 cloves garlic, smashed

10 black peppercorns

2 bay leaves

Fresh herbs such as thyme or rosemary sprigs (optional)

Filtered water

1. If making beef broth: Preheat the oven to 400°F. Place the beef bones on a heavy rimmed baking sheet. Brush them with the tomato paste. Roast until they are well browned, about 30 minutes.

2. For all broths: Combine the bones (beef and/or poultry), vegetable scraps, garlic, peppercorns, bay leaves, and herbs (if using) in a large stockpot, slow cooker, or Instant Pot. Cover completely with filtered water. Cook according to one of the following methods.

STOVETOP: Bring the water to a boil over high heat, then reduce the temperature so the water is just lightly simmering. Simmer for several hours—the longer the better—keeping an eye on the water level. Add more water if it gets too low.

SLOW COOKER: Cover and cook on low (undisturbed) for at least 8 hours, but longer is better. You can cook it for 24 hours or more.

INSTANT POT: Press the Manual button and set the cook time to 120 minutes. When the time is up, turn off the Instant Pot and allow the pressure to release naturally.

recipe continues

MACRONUTRIENTS PER 1 CUP (CHICKEN BONE BROTH)
CALORIES: 86
FAT: 3 G/26 CALORIES
CARBOHYDRATE: 9 G/ 34 CALORIES
PROTEIN: 6 G/24 CALORIES

MACRONUTRIENTS PER 1 CUP (BEEF BONE BROTH)
CALORIES: 31
FAT: <1 G/2 CALORIES
CARBOHYDRATE: 3 G/ 12 CALORIES
PROTEIN: 5 G/19 CALORIES

3. To rapidly cool the broth, fill your kitchen sink with ice water. Place a metal bowl in the ice water and place a metal sieve or colander over the bowl. Carefully strain the hot broth into the bowl (discard the solids). Allow it to chill for about 15 minutes, stirring occasionally.

4. Optional: Strain the broth again through a fine-mesh sieve into a spouted measuring cup. Pour the broth into mason jars, leaving about 1 inch of headspace. Secure the lids and place the jars immediately in the refrigerator or freezer. (Alternatively, you can pour the broth into ice cube trays or silicone molds and freeze it.) Use refrigerated broth within a few days.

BASIC CAULIFLOWER RICE

Cauliflower rice is something one rarely heard about outside primal/paleo circles just a few years ago, and now it seems like every grocery store carries priced cauliflower in the produce and freezer sections. These products are great timesavers, although cauliflower rice is also easy to make yourself. Once you have mastered cauliflower rice, there are endless ways you can turn this simple side dish into something even more special. Double this basic recipe to feed a bigger group or so you can have a ready-made supply to include in a recipe.

SERVES 4

4   cups riced cauliflower (about 14 ounces)

2   tablespoons avocado oil

Sea salt

MACRONUTRIENTS PER SERVING

CALORIES: 85

FAT: 7 G/64 CALORIES

CARBOHYDRATE: 5 G/ 20 CALORIES

PROTEIN: 2 G/8 CALORIES

Mix it up! Check out the recipes for Triple-Coconut Cauliflower Rice (page 165) and Keto Shrimp Fried Rice (page 115).

BROILER METHOD (PREFERRED)

1. Position an oven rack 2 to 3 inches from the broiler. Preheat the broiler to low.

2. In a bowl, combine the cauliflower, oil, and ½ teaspoon salt, stirring well to coat the cauliflower with the oil. Spread the cauliflower evenly on a heavy rimmed baking sheet.

3. Place the cauliflower under the hot broiler and broil for 4 minutes, keeping an eye on it to make sure it isn't burning. The edges should begin to brown. Remove the pan from the oven and stir the cauliflower. Spread it evenly in the pan again, and return it to the oven for 2 more minutes. Remove it from the oven and transfer the cauliflower rice to a serving bowl. Taste and adjust the salt if desired.

STOVETOP METHOD

1. In a large skillet or wok, heat the avocado oil over medium heat. Add the cauliflower and ½ teaspoon salt, and stir well. Stir-fry for about 3 minutes.

2. Cover and cook until tender, 3 to 5 minutes longer. Taste and adjust the salt if desired.

NUT MILK

Nut milk is one of those things that you can buy in the store, but once you make it yourself, you may never go back to store-bought. Homemade is much tastier and free from any objectionable added ingredients (especially sweeteners, which are prominent in many products—read labels carefully!). Nut milk is an excellent macronutrient-balanced base for smoothies. It also makes a great alternative for your morning coffee (if you are trying to get away from high-fat coffee bombs in the morning) or for Creamy Keto Hot Chocolate (page 248).

MAKES 4 CUPS

1	cup raw nuts (almonds, hazelnuts, cashews, pecans, or macadamias)
3 to 4	cups filtered water, plus more for soaking

ADD-INS (OPTIONAL)

1	teaspoon vanilla extract
¼	teaspoon sea salt
½	teaspoon ground cinnamon
	Keto-friendly sweetener, to taste

MACRONUTRIENTS PER 1 CUP

CALORIES: 36

FAT: 3 G/26 CALORIES

CARBOHYDRATE: 1 G/ 6 CALORIES

PROTEIN: 1 G/6 CALORIES

1. Place the nuts in a glass bowl or jar and cover entirely with filtered water. Soak the nuts at room temperature for at least 4 hours, but preferably 8 hours or overnight.

2. Drain and rinse the nuts. Place the soaked nuts in a high-powered blender with 3 to 4 cups fresh filtered water (use 4 cups if the capacity of your blender allows, but less if needed so as not to overfill it). Blend on high until very smooth.

3. Strain the nut milk through a nut milk bag (see Note) or a clean kitchen towel into a bowl. Squeeze the pulp to release as much milk as possible.

4. If you are adding any of the optional ingredients, rinse out the blender, add the milk and optional ingredients, and blend until smooth.

5. Transfer the nut milk to an airtight container and refrigerate. Use within 5 days.

Note: Nut milk bags are fine-mesh bags that are incredibly useful to have if you make nut milk often. Check to see if your natural foods store stocks them, or you can find them online. Save the nut pulp to use in smoothies, bread, or recipes such as the Nut Pulp Rolls or Hamburger Buns (page 224). If you have a food dehydrator, you can also dehydrate it to make nut meal.

BIGASS SALAD

As readers of my blog know already, the centerpiece of my primal eating strategy is a midday Bigass Salad (search YouTube for "Mark Sisson Bigass Steak Salad" to see a preparation in action). You can eat a different Bigass Salad every day of the week, packed with colorful veggies, protein, and healthy fats, and never get bored thanks to the endless possibilities. Following is a basic recipe that you can adjust for size or different ingredients as desired.

MAKES I BIGASS SALAD

4	cups lettuce or mixed salad greens (5 to 6 ounces), chopped
2	cups assorted sliced/chopped veggies (mushrooms, bell peppers, zucchini, carrots, broccoli, beets, etc.)
¼	cup shredded cheese
¼	cup nuts (walnuts, pecans, almonds)
2	tablespoons sunflower or pumpkin seeds
4 to 5	ounces protein of choice (canned tuna or sardines; cooked chicken, turkey, or steak)
1	hard-boiled egg, sliced
½ to 1	avocado, sliced
2	tablespoons of your favorite keto-friendly dressing (ensure it's free from refined high polyunsaturated vegetable oils, such as canola, soybean, sunflower, and the like)

1. In a large bowl, layer the lettuce, veggies, and cheese. If you want, toss these ingredients with half the dressing.

2. Sprinkle the nuts and seeds on top, followed by your protein of choice. Arrange the sliced egg and avocado on top, and drizzle everything with the remaining dressing. Eat immediately.

Note: If you are packing your salad ahead of time, leave the dressing off, and keep the nuts and seeds separate from the rest of the ingredients until just before eating.

MACRONUTRIENTS PER SERVING*

CALORIES: 907

FAT: 64 G/578 CALORIES

CARBOHYDRATE: 27 G/109 CALORIES

PROTEIN: 60 G/241 CALORIES

* Macros vary according to exact ingredients chosen. The numbers here are for a Bigass Salad with ½ cup each raw mushrooms and zucchini, 1 cup broccoli florets, 4 ounces skin-on chicken breast, and 2 tablespoons Primal Kitchen Greek Dressing.

BREAKFAST

Remember, traditional breakfast foods are just a cultural norm, but you can get creative with any food that you choose to break your overnight fast. Other recipes in the book that make a great first meal of the day are:

- Turnip Kohlrabi Gratin (page 188)—like cheesy breakfast potatoes!
- Taco Turkey Burgers (page 114)
- One-Pan Chicken and Veggies (page 132)
- Pan-Seared Salmon with Quick Hollandaise and Crispy Capers (page 135)
- Creamy Sautéed Liver (yes, really!) (page 129)
- Tuna Cakes (page 147)
- Offal Bacon Burgers (page 145)
- Chopped Liver (page 210)
- Berry Blintzes (page 228)
- Spaghetti Squash Carbonara (page 190)
- Avocado Stuffed with Salmon Salad (page 81)
- Handheld Chef Salad (page 103)

Truly, there isn't a recipe in this book that wouldn't be great to eat at any time of the day! Plus, breaking a fast with last night's leftovers saves a ton of time. Maybe freeing yourself from the idea of "breakfast foods" is the ultimate food freedom?

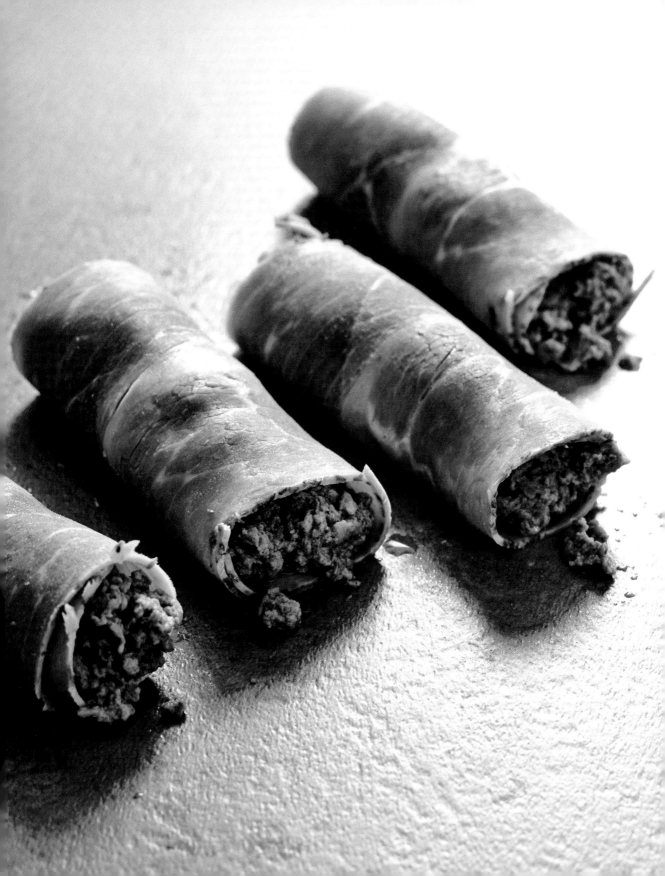

GREEN EGGS AND HAM

A breakfast to make Dr. Seuss proud. Trying to encourage your kids to eat a more primal-aligned diet? Start here.

SERVES 2

1½ cups packed baby spinach

3 tablespoons heavy whipping cream or full-fat coconut milk

3 large eggs

Pinch of sea salt

Pinch of ground black pepper

1 tablespoon unsalted butter or ghee

4 slices deli ham (about 4 ounces)

MACRONUTRIENTS PER SERVING
CALORIES: 303
FAT: 23 G/209 CALORIES
CARBOHYDRATE: 3 G/ 11 CALORIES
PROTEIN: 21 G/85 CALORIES

1. In a blender or small food processor, combine the spinach and cream and blend until the spinach is finely chopped, about 20 seconds. If needed, scrape down the sides of the blender and blend another 5 to 10 seconds.

2. Scrape down the sides of the blender again. Add the eggs, salt, and pepper and pulse until just combined.

3. In a medium skillet, heat the butter over medium heat. Pour the egg mixture into the pan and cook, stirring frequently, to scramble the eggs to your preferred doneness.

4. Meanwhile, place the ham on a microwave-safe plate and microwave on high for 15 seconds.

5. When the eggs are set, divide the egg mixture evenly among the 4 slices of ham. Roll each slice like a burrito around the eggs and secure with a toothpick. Serve immediately.

Mix it up!
- Try this recipe with baby kale or Swiss chard instead of spinach.
- Top the eggs with shredded white cheddar cheese.
- Add sliced avocados to the ham rolls.

BIGASS BREAKFAST SALAD WITH BACON DRESSING

One big difference between how we primal/keto folks eat and how the average SAD eater starts their day is that we love to incorporate big servings of colorful veggies into our first meal of the day. Whether that means an omelet or a Bigass Breakfast Salad, starting your day with some veggies gets you off on the right foot.

SERVES 2

4 slices sugar-free bacon

½ cup sliced mushrooms

¼ cup diced yellow or red bell pepper

4 large eggs

¼ teaspoon sea salt

⅛ teaspoon ground black pepper, plus more to taste

4 cups spring mix or baby spinach (6 ounces)

½ cup cherry tomatoes, halved

1 medium avocado, diced

¼ cup shredded cheddar cheese (optional)

FOR THE DRESSING

2 tablespoons bacon fat

1 tablespoon apple cider vinegar

2 teaspoons Dijon mustard

1. In a medium skillet, cook the bacon over medium heat until crispy, about 3 minutes. Transfer the bacon to a plate.

2. Pour off all but about 1 tablespoon of the bacon fat from the skillet into a small bowl. Measure out 2 tablespoons and set aside for the dressing. (Save any remaining bacon fat for use in another recipe.)

3. In the same skillet, add the mushrooms and bell pepper. Sauté over medium heat until the vegetables start to soften, about 4 minutes.

OPTION 1: Push the vegetables to the sides of the pan and crack the eggs into the center. Sprinkle the eggs with the salt and pepper. Cook for 3 minutes on the first side, then flip the eggs and cook until yolks reach the desired firmness: about 1 more minute for over-easy, 2 more minutes for over-medium, 3 more minutes for over-well.

OPTION 2: Lightly beat the eggs in a small bowl. Pour the beaten eggs over the vegetables in the skillet and season with the salt and pepper. Scramble the eggs and vegetables together until the eggs are just set, about 3 minutes.

4. Meanwhile, divide the spring mix, cherry tomatoes, and avocado between two bowls. Crumble 2 pieces of bacon over each salad.

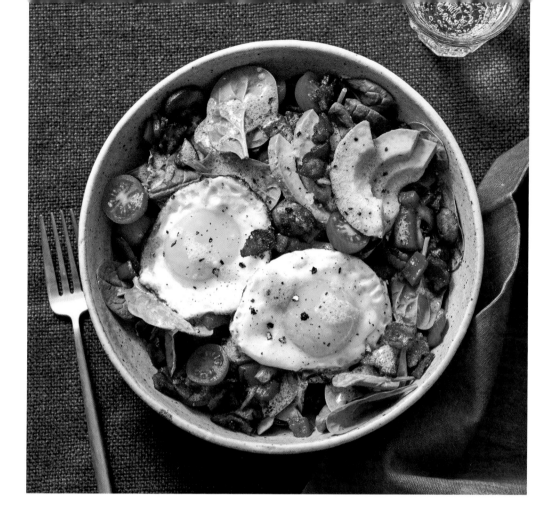

MACRONUTRIENTS PER SERVING
(NO CHEESE)

CALORIES: 554

FAT: 46 G/418 CALORIES

CARBOHYDRATE: 15 G/
60 CALORIES

PROTEIN: 23 G/91 CALORIES

MACRONUTRIENTS PER SERVING
(WITH CHEESE)

CALORIES: 609

FAT: 51 G/458 CALORIES

CARBOHYDRATE: 15 G/
62 CALORIES

PROTEIN: 26 G/105 CALORIES

5. For the dressing: In a small bowl, whisk together the 2 tablespoons reserved bacon fat, apple cider vinegar, and mustard. Drizzle the dressing over the salads.

6. When the eggs are cooked to your liking, place them on top of the salads. If desired, sprinkle with cheddar and crack a bit of black pepper over the top of each salad. Serve immediately.

TIP: To save time in the morning, make the crumbled bacon and the dressing the night before, and chop the veggies. Store everything in the refrigerator overnight. The next morning, warm the bacon and the dressing in the microwave for 15 to 30 seconds while you cook your eggs.

EASY CHEESY BAKED EGGS

You can get these in the oven quickly in the morning and let them bake while you get ready for your day; you can also make them ahead and reheat them. The recipe can easily be doubled, tripled, or more if you are serving lots of people, and you can tweak it in tons of ways to make it something slightly different each time. Serve them with a side of sugar-free bacon or sausage, a dollop of sour cream and guacamole, and some salsa for a quick and easy complete breakfast.

SERVES 4

2 tablespoons butter, at room temperature, or Primal Kitchen Avocado Oil Spray

8 large eggs

½ teaspoon sea salt

½ teaspoon ground black pepper

½ cup shredded sharp cheddar cheese

¼ cup shredded Parmesan cheese

MACRONUTRIENTS PER SERVING (2 EGGS)

CALORIES: 282

FAT: 22 G/198 CALORIES

CARBOHYDRATE: 2 G/ 6 CALORIES

PROTEIN: 18 G/72 CALORIES

1. Preheat the oven to 350°F. Grease 8 cups of a muffin tin with the butter (or spray with oil), making sure to get the sides of the cups because the eggs will rise. (Silicone muffin cups work great for this recipe.)

2. Crack 1 egg into each cup and add a dash of salt and pepper to each. Use a fork to give each egg a quick stir to break the yolk. It is not necessary to mix the egg white and yolk completely.

3. Add 1 tablespoon shredded cheddar to each cup and stir again. Top each egg with ½ tablespoon Parmesan.

4. Bake until the eggs are completely set, 17 to 20 minutes. Remove them from the oven. Let them cool for a few minutes, then carefully remove the eggs from the cups. These can be served immediately or stored in the refrigerator in an airtight container to be reheated later.

Mix it up!
- Add ¼ teaspoon Italian Seasoning Blend (page 254) or turmeric to each egg.
- Use different types of cheese: Try goat cheese instead of Parmesan, or pepper jack instead of cheddar, for example.
- Add cooked meat and veggies. (This is a great way to use up leftover roasted vegetables!)

BLUEBERRIES AND CREAM EGGS

If you used to love blueberry pancakes in your pre-primal, pre-keto days, this is the recipe for you! It sounds weird on paper, but you will be hooked once you try it.

SERVES 2

4   large eggs

2   tablespoons vanilla-flavored protein or collagen powder

¼   cup heavy whipping cream or full-fat coconut milk

1   teaspoon vanilla extract

¼   teaspoon kosher salt

¼   cup blueberries

1   tablespoon raw cacao butter or unsalted butter

2   tablespoons coconut butter, at room temperature

1. In a small bowl, mix together the eggs, protein powder, cream, vanilla, and salt. Stir until no lumps remain, then lightly beat for another 20 to 30 seconds. Stir in the blueberries.

2. In a small saucepan, melt the cacao butter over low heat. When it is just melted, stir in the coconut butter. As soon as the coconut butter is incorporated, pour the egg mixture into the saucepan. Cook, stirring every 30 seconds or so, until the eggs are just set, 2 to 3 minutes. Cook for an additional minute if you want more-well-done eggs. Transfer to two plates and enjoy warm.

MACRONUTRIENTS PER SERVING*

CALORIES: 471

FAT: 40 G/361 CALORIES

CARBOHYDRATE: 10 G/ 40 CALORIES

PROTEIN: 19 G/76 CALORIES

* Macros based on using Primal Kitchen Vanilla Coconut Collagen Fuel.

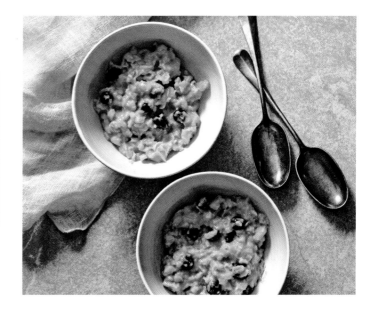

OVERNIGHT NUTTY CHOCOLATE CHIA PUDDING

Overnight Chai Chia Breakfast Pudding was one of the most popular recipes in *The Keto Reset Diet*, but this recipe will give it a run for its money. This version is heartier than its *TKRD* cousin thanks to the addition of chopped nuts and cacao nibs. Think of it as a cross between chia pudding and overnight oats.

SERVES 2

1	cup unsweetened nut milk (see Note), homemade (page 38) or store-bought
2	tablespoons chia seeds
⅓	cup walnut or pecan pieces
1	tablespoon cacao nibs
1	tablespoon cacao powder
1	teaspoon vanilla extract
¼	teaspoon ground cinnamon
⅛	teaspoon sea salt
8 to 10	drops liquid stevia, to taste, or keto-friendly sweetener of choice
2	tablespoons collagen peptides (optional)

1. In a small bowl, stir together the nut milk, chia seeds, nuts, cacao nibs, cacao powder, vanilla, cinnamon, and salt. Add half the sweetener and taste the liquid. Increase the amount of sweetener if you choose.

2. Divide the mixture between two small jars or glass bowls. If using, add 1 tablespoon collagen peptides to each and stir well. Cover the jars tightly and give them a gentle shake. Refrigerate overnight.

3. In the morning, give the chia puddings a good stir. You can eat them cold, let them come to room temperature, or heat them in the microwave. They will keep for several days in the refrigerator.

Note: If you are nut-free, use ¾ cup + 2 tablespoons full-fat coconut milk or heavy whipping cream diluted with 2 tablespoons water (to achieve the same consistency) instead of nut milk.

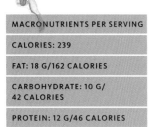

MACRONUTRIENTS PER SERVING

CALORIES: 239

FAT: 18 G/162 CALORIES

CARBOHYDRATE: 10 G/ 42 CALORIES

PROTEIN: 12 G/46 CALORIES

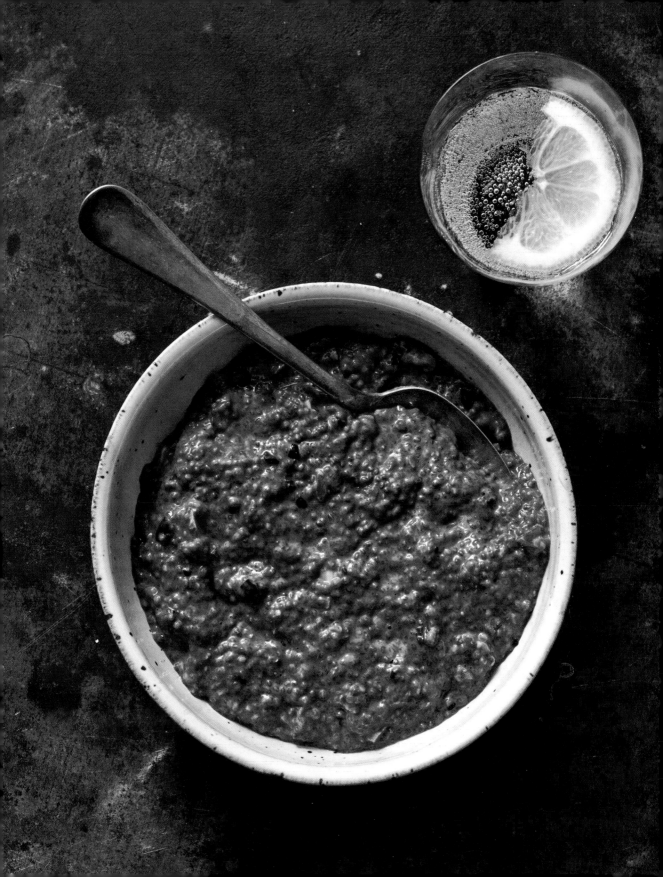

SAUSAGE GRAVY

If you thought you couldn't enjoy biscuits and gravy on keto, think again! Pair this recipe with the Basic Biscuits (page 223). Also think outside the biscuit box. This gravy is equally great over scrambled eggs, sautéed green beans, or with Keto Home Fries with Greens (page 66).

SERVES 6

- 1 pound bulk sugar-free sausage (breakfast or other mild flavor)
- 1 tablespoon ghee or coconut oil
- 1 tablespoon coconut flour, sifted
- 1 (13.5-ounce) can full-fat coconut milk
- ½ teaspoon garlic powder

  Sea salt and ground black pepper

1. Heat a medium skillet over medium-high heat. Add the sausage and break it up with a fork. Cook until no pink remains, 10 to 12 minutes.

2. Add the ghee and stir the sausage until the ghee is fully melted. Sprinkle the coconut flour over the sausage. Stir to evenly distribute the coconut flour into the meat.

3. Add the coconut milk, garlic powder, and ½ teaspoon each salt and pepper. Stir well. Allow the mixture to come to a boil, then gently boil, stirring frequently until thickened, about 7 minutes. Taste and adjust the salt and pepper as needed, then serve immediately.

MACRONUTRIENTS PER SERVING
CALORIES: 387
FAT: 35 G/319 CALORIES
CARBOHYDRATE: 4 G/ 15 CALORIES
PROTEIN: 15 G/60 CALORIES

HEARTY COCONUT N'OATMEAL

One of the things that has to go when you switch from a SAD to a primal or keto eating style is oatmeal, but it turns out that hemp hearts make a very decent substitute. Hemp hearts (a.k.a. hulled hemp seeds) are also a great plant-based source of omega-3 and omega-6 fatty acids, protein, and fiber.

SERVES 2

1   cup full-fat coconut milk

½   cup hemp hearts

¼   cup unsweetened finely shredded coconut

2   teaspoons raw cacao butter or coconut oil

¼   teaspoon vanilla extract

⅛   teaspoon ground cardamom

     Pinch of sea salt

TOPPINGS (OPTIONAL)

Butter

Coconut butter

Heavy whipping cream

Nut or seed butter

In a saucepan, combine the coconut milk, hemp hearts, coconut, cacao butter, vanilla, cardamom, and salt and heat over medium until it just begins to bubble, about 2 minutes. Reduce the heat to low and cook, just simmering, for about 10 minutes. If the mixture starts to get too thick, add a tablespoon of water. Transfer to two bowls and top with optional toppings.

MACRONUTRIENTS PER SERVING
(NO OPTIONAL TOPPINGS)

CALORIES: 518

FAT: 45 G/404 CALORIES

CARBOHYDRATE: 10 G/
38 CALORIES

PROTEIN: 16 G/62 CALORIES

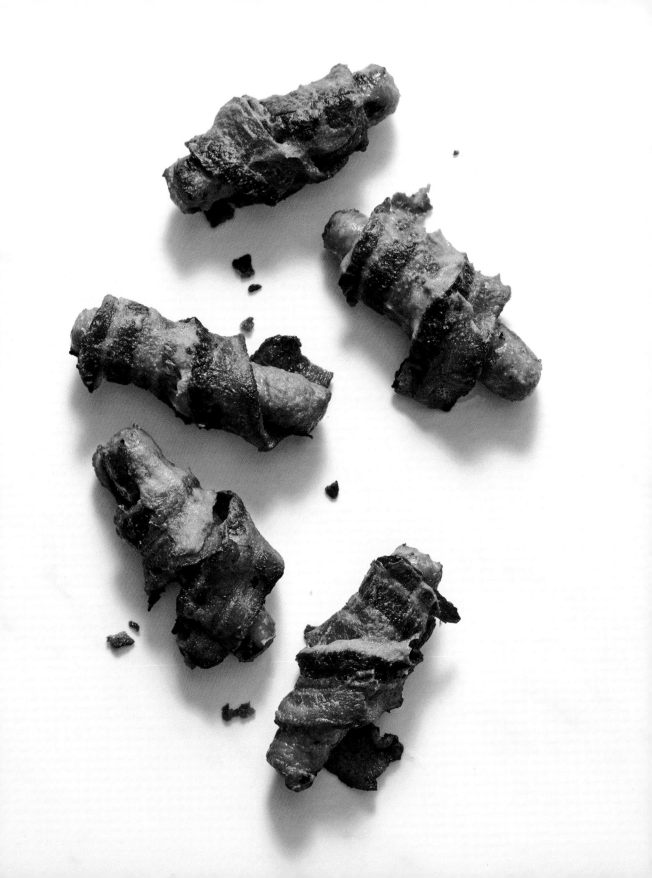

BACON-WRAPPED SAUSAGE

Sure, you can eat bacon and sausage side by side, but have you eaten them together?? This fun dish is perfect for your next keto brunch. Don't skip the Dijon mustard.

SERVES 4

8 links sugar-free breakfast sausage

8 slices sugar-free bacon

1½ teaspoons Dijon mustard

MACRONUTRIENTS PER SERVING (2 SAUSAGES)

CALORIES: 252

FAT: 22 G/202 CALORIES

CARBOHYDRATE: 1 G/ 2 CALORIES

PROTEIN: 12 G/46 CALORIES

1. Heat a large skillet over medium heat. In two batches, cook the bacon, flipping once, until cooked but still pliable, about 5 minutes. Place the cooked bacon on a plate lined with paper towel and set aside.

2. Pour most of the fat out of the skillet into a small jar and set aside. Add the breakfast sausage to the pan and cook according to package directions. Transfer the cooked sausage to paper towels to drain and cool slightly.

3. When cool enough to handle, working carefully, wrap one piece of bacon around each sausage link on a diagonal so that the sausage is nearly covered by bacon. Secure the end with a toothpick. Arrange the sausages on a broilerproof pan.

4. Position an oven rack 4 to 6 inches from the broiler. Preheat the broiler to low.

5. In a small glass bowl, stir together the mustard and 1 teaspoon of the reserved bacon fat. Use a pastry brush to dab some of the mixture over the top of the sausages.

6. Broil the sausages until the bacon is crispy, about 2 minutes, watching to make sure they don't burn. Remove the sausages and flip them. Dab the second side with the mustard mixture and return them to the broiler for about 30 seconds more.

7. If desired, transfer the sausages to a plate lined with paper towel to drain. Allow them to cool for a few minutes, remove the toothpicks, and serve warm.

CREAM CHEESE PANCAKES

You won't believe how good these are considering they only have two ingredients! Start with the basic recipe and then let your creative juices flow. What follows are two ways you can modify the basic recipe into something even more interesting.

MAKES SIX
4-INCH PANCAKES
/ SERVES 2

2 ounces full-fat cream cheese

2 large eggs

1½ teaspoons butter

MACRONUTRIENTS PER SERVING
(3 PANCAKES)

CALORIES: 177

FAT: 16 G/141 CALORIES

CARBOHYDRATE: 2 G/
6 CALORIES

PROTEIN: 8 G/30 CALORIES

1. Heat a small skillet (6½-inch diameter is ideal) over medium-low to low heat for 3 to 4 minutes. Meanwhile, in a blender, combine the cream cheese and eggs and blend until smooth.

2. Melt ¼ teaspoon butter in the center of the skillet and swirl to coat. Pour about 2 tablespoons of batter into the pan using a circular motion to spread the batter a bit thinner than a traditional pancake and gently swirl the pan. Cook for 90 seconds on the first side. Carefully flip (see Tip) and cook 30 seconds on the other side. Remove to a plate and repeat with the rest of the batter, greasing the pan with butter before cooking each pancake.

TIP: If the pancakes tear, make sure your heat is set low and try cooking an additional 15 seconds on the first side. Don't worry, you can still use them even if they tear!

HAM AND GRUYÈRE PANCAKES

2　ounces full-fat cream cheese

2　large eggs

1½　teaspoons butter

3　slices deli ham, halved

¾　cup shredded Gruyère cheese

MACRONUTRIENTS PER SERVING
(3 PANCAKES)

CALORIES: 568

FAT: 44 G/399 CALORIES

CARBOHYDRATE: 2 G/
9 CALORIES

PROTEIN: 39 G/156 CALORIES

1. Heat a small skillet (6½-inch diameter is ideal) over medium-low to low heat for 3 to 4 minutes. Meanwhile, in a blender, combine the cream cheese and eggs and blend until smooth.

2. Melt a generous ¼ teaspoon butter in the center of the skillet and swirl to coat. Pour about 2 tablespoons of batter into the pan using a circular motion to spread the batter a bit thinner than a traditional pancake and gently swirl the pan. (You can also use the back of a spoon to gently spread out the batter.) Cook for 90 seconds on the first side. Carefully flip (see Tip, opposite) and cook 30 seconds on the other side. Remove to a plate and repeat with the rest of the batter, greasing the pan with butter before cooking each pancake.

3. Remove the pan from the heat. Place a half slice of ham and 2 tablespoons of shredded cheese on each pancake, and fold in half to cover the filling. Place the folded pancakes back in the warm pan, stacking as necessary, and cover the pan. Let the pancakes sit covered for a minute to melt the cheese. If needed, briefly turn the burner back on warm.

4. Serve the pancakes warm.

BERRY LEMON RICOTTA CREPES

MAKES SIX
4-INCH PANCAKES
/ SERVES 2

FOR THE BERRY FILLING

½ cup berries, any variety

Grated zest and juice of 1 Meyer lemon or 1 small regular lemon

1 tablespoon water

¼ teaspoon vanilla extract

1 to 2 drops liquid stevia, or other keto-friendly sweetener (optional)

FOR THE CREPE BATTER

2 large eggs

1 ounce full-fat cream cheese

2 tablespoons whole-milk ricotta cheese

¼ teaspoon vanilla extract

TO COOK AND ASSEMBLE

2 teaspoons unsalted butter + 6 teaspoons unsalted butter for topping

¼ cup whole-milk ricotta cheese

MACRONUTRIENTS PER SERVING (3 PANCAKES)

CALORIES: 329

FAT: 27 G/243 CALORIES

CARBOHYDRATE: 10 G/ 40 CALORIES

PROTEIN: 13 G/52 CALORIES

1. For the berry filling: In a small saucepan, combine the berries, lemon zest, lemon juice, water, and vanilla and heat over medium heat. When it starts to bubble, turn the heat down as low as possible and simmer gently until the berries break down, 5 minutes. Taste the berry filling and decide if you want to add any sweetener.

2. Heat a small skillet (6½-inch diameter is ideal) over medium-low to low heat for 3 to 4 minutes.

3. Meanwhile, for the crepe batter: In a blender, combine the eggs, cream cheese, ricotta, and vanilla and blend until smooth.

4. To cook the crepes: Melt a generous ¼ teaspoon butter in the center of the skillet and swirl to coat. Pour about 2 tablespoons of batter into the pan using a circular motion to spread the batter a bit thinner than a traditional pancake and gently swirl the pan. (You can also use the back of a spoon to gently spread out the batter.) Cook for 90 seconds on the first side. Carefully flip (see Tip, page 54) and cook 30 seconds on the other side. Remove to a plate and repeat with the rest of the batter, greasing the pan with butter before cooking each crepe. Keep the skillet at the ready, but off the stove.

5. To assemble: Working with one crepe at a time, use the back of a spoon to spread 2 teaspoons ricotta down the middle of the crepe. Spoon about 2 teaspoons of the berry filling over the ricotta. Roll up the crepe and place it seam side down in the pan to keep warm (the residual heat of the pan will do this). Repeat for the remaining crepes. To serve, place the crepes seam side down on plates and top with each with 1 teaspoon butter.

GREEK FRITTATA WITH TZATZIKI

This frittata has all the flavors of your favorite Greek salad. Olives and eggs might seem like an unusual combo, but they actually pair nicely. To save time, you can prepare the tzatziki the night before. Just give it a good stir before serving.

SERVES 4

1 tablespoon bacon fat, lard, tallow, or fat of choice

8 ounces ground lamb

1 teaspoon Greek Seasoning Blend (page 253)

½ teaspoon sea salt

1 clove garlic, minced

6 large eggs

¼ teaspoon ground black pepper

½ cup diced zucchini

½ cup grape tomatoes, halved

1 cup baby spinach

¼ cup kalamata olives, chopped

1 to 2 tablespoons water or broth (optional)

⅔ cup crumbled feta cheese

Tzatziki Sauce (recipe follows), for serving

MACRONUTRIENTS PER SERVING

CALORIES: 556

FAT: 42 G/378 CALORIES

CARBOHYDRATE: 10 G/40 CALORIES

PROTEIN: 34 G/136 CALORIES

1. In a 10-inch skillet, warm the fat over medium-high heat. Crumble the ground lamb into the skillet. Cook, stirring occasionally and breaking up the meat with a spoon or meat chopper, for 3 minutes. Stir in ½ teaspoon of the Greek seasoning, ¼ teaspoon of the salt, and the garlic and cook until the lamb is almost cooked through, 3 to 5 minutes.

2. While the meat is cooking, in a bowl, lightly beat the eggs. Whisk in the remaining ½ teaspoon Greek seasoning, ¼ teaspoon salt, and the pepper. Set aside.

3. If the skillet is dry, add some additional fat. Stir in the zucchini, tomatoes, and spinach and cook until zucchini becomes soft but not mushy, 3 to 4 minutes. Stir in the olives. If needed, use the water to deglaze the pan, scraping up any browned bits stuck to the bottom.

4. Reduce the heat to medium. Pour in the egg mixture. Stir in half the feta cheese. Allow the eggs to cook until the egg mixture is about halfway set, about 4 minutes. While they cook, use a silicone spatula to gently pull the eggs away from the sides of the pan. Do not scramble the eggs, but allow some of the raw egg mixture on top to pour into the open space you created with the spatula.

recipe continues

5. When the egg mixture is about halfway set, sprinkle the remaining feta cheese on top. Reduce the heat to medium-low and cover the skillet. Allow the frittata to cook undisturbed for 5 minutes.

6. Check the frittata. You will know it is done when it puffs up and the eggs no longer appear wet in the center. Remove the pan from the heat and allow it to sit for a few minutes. Run a sharp knife around the edge of the frittata.

7. Cut the frittata into wedges and use a spatula to carefully remove it from the pan. Serve warm with the tzatziki on the side.

TZATZIKI SAUCE

MAKES ABOUT 1 CUP

½   English cucumber, striped (lightly peeled) and grated

Kosher salt

1   cup plain full-fat Greek yogurt, coconut milk yogurt, or almond milk yogurt

2   teaspoons fresh lemon juice

2   cloves garlic, pressed or finely minced

Ground black pepper

Place the grated cucumber in a sieve set over a bowl. Sprinkle with ¼ teaspoon kosher salt, stir, and set aside for 10 minutes. Use a spatula or the back of a large spoon to press as much liquid as possible out of the grated cucumber. Stir and press again. Repeat until no more liquid is coming out. Transfer the cucumber to a small bowl and stir in the yogurt, lemon juice, garlic, and ¼ teaspoon pepper. Taste and adjust the salt and pepper. Place it in the refrigerator until ready to serve.

Note: This tzatziki recipe calls for only half a cucumber because a higher yogurt-to-vegetable ratio is nice for topping a frittata. Feel free to use more cucumber in yours if you prefer (adjust the salt accordingly).

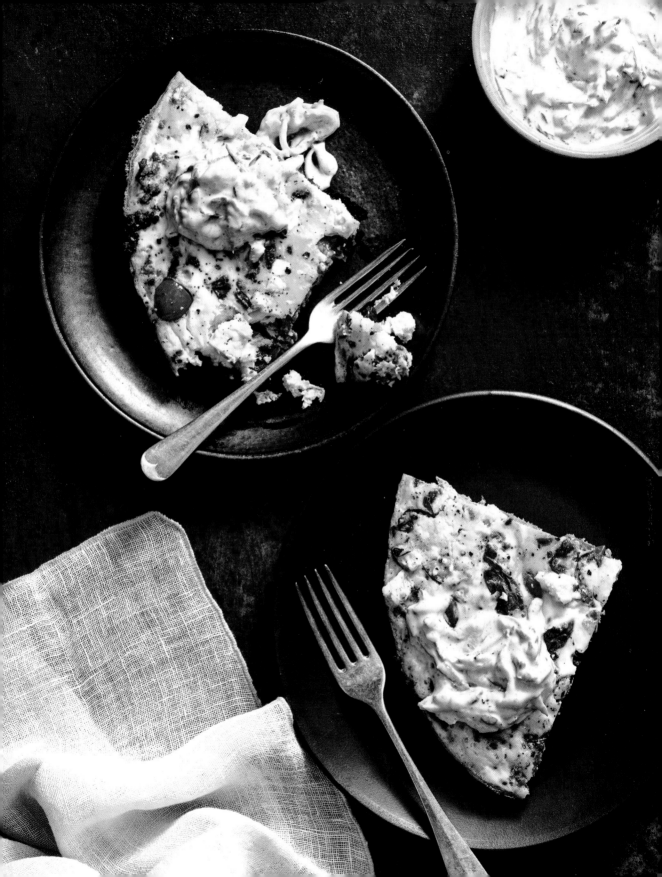

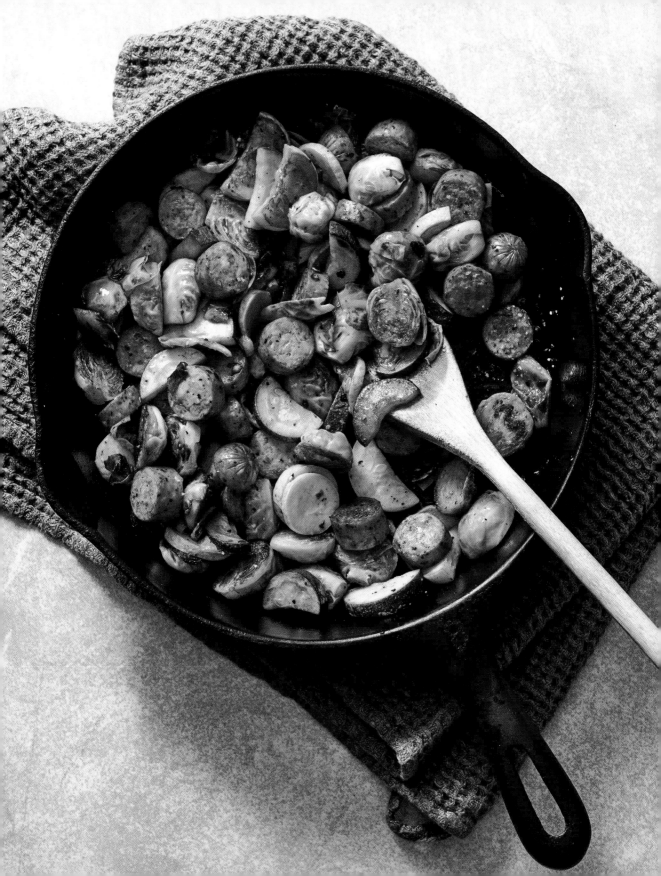

SAUSAGE AND VEGGIE SKILLET

Many people struggle to find nonegg options that still feel "breakfasty" on keto. While this recipe would certainly be delicious at any time of day, you can use (sugar-free) breakfast sausage to make it feel like a more traditional "breakfast food." Experiment with using chorizo, Italian, or any other flavor of pork or chicken sausage.

SERVES 2

¼ cup avocado oil

6 ounces Brussels sprouts, trimmed and halved
Sea salt

6 ounces fully cooked sugar-free chicken sausage, cut into bite-size pieces

1 small zucchini, quartered lengthwise and cut crosswise into ¼-inch slices

1 small yellow squash, halved lengthwise and cut into ¼-inch slices

1 tablespoon salted butter

2 tablespoons avocado oil–based dressing (optional), such as Caesar, Italian, or balsamic vinaigrette

MACRONUTRIENTS PER SERVING*

CALORIES: 543

FAT: 48 G/435 CALORIES

CARBOHYDRATE: 11 G/ 43 CALORIES

PROTEIN: 21 G/83 CALORIES

* Macros based on using Primal Kitchen Caesar Dressing.

1. Pour the avocado oil into a large, COLD skillet. Place the Brussels sprouts in the pan cut side down and place a lid on the pan. Turn the heat to medium and cook undisturbed for 5 minutes. Uncover and, without disturbing the Brussels sprouts, cook 2 minutes more. Sprinkle with ½ teaspoon salt and stir.

2. Push the Brussels sprouts to the side of the pan and slide the pan so that the Brussels sprouts are off direct heat. Add the sausage to the empty space and cook, stirring frequently, until the sausage is just warmed through, 2 minutes. (If your pan is not large enough, you can remove the Brussels sprouts to a separate bowl for this step.)

3. Add the zucchini, squash, and butter to the sausage. Stir all the contents of the pan, including the Brussels sprouts, together. Add the dressing (if using) and stir well, scraping up any browned bits stuck to the bottom of the pan. (If you are not using the dressing, you can deglaze the pan with a couple tablespoons of water or bone broth.) Cook until the zucchini and squash are just tender, about 2 minutes more. Taste and adjust the salt. Serve immediately.

BLANCHED AND SAUTÉED VEGETABLES WITH QUICK HOLLANDAISE

I'm a big proponent of eating a big serving of vegetables at breakfast. This dish comes together quickly if you prep the vegetables and even make the hollandaise the night before.

SERVES 4

1 tablespoon + ½ teaspoon kosher salt

1 large broccoli crown, cut into small florets (about 3 cups)

1 bunch asparagus, woody ends cut off, cut on a diagonal into 1½-inch lengths

¼ pound green beans, ends trimmed, halved

2 tablespoons bacon fat, butter, or ghee, or fat of choice

¼ teaspoon ground black pepper

Quick Hollandaise (page 257)

8 slices sugar-free bacon, cooked and crumbled

1. In a large stockpot, bring 10 cups water and 1 tablespoon kosher salt to a rolling boil. Fill a large bowl with ice water.

2. Add the broccoli, asparagus, and beans to the boiling water and set a timer for 2 minutes.

3. Use a slotted spoon or a fine-mesh sieve to remove the vegetables from the boiling water and transfer them to the ice bath. Allow the vegetables to chill for 2 minutes. Drain them very well, shaking off all the excess water, and pat the vegetables dry with a clean kitchen towel.

4. In a large skillet or wok, heat the fat over medium heat. Carefully add the vegetables (watch for splatter), season with the ½ teaspoon kosher salt and the pepper, and sauté until the vegetables are crisp-tender, 3 to 5 minutes.

5. Divide the vegetables among four serving bowls. Top each with 3 tablespoons hollandaise. Sprinkle with the bacon and serve warm.

MACRONUTRIENTS PER SERVING

CALORIES: 438

FAT: 41 G/365 CALORIES

CARBOHYDRATE: 10 G/ 38 CALORIES

PROTEIN: 12 G/49 CALORIES

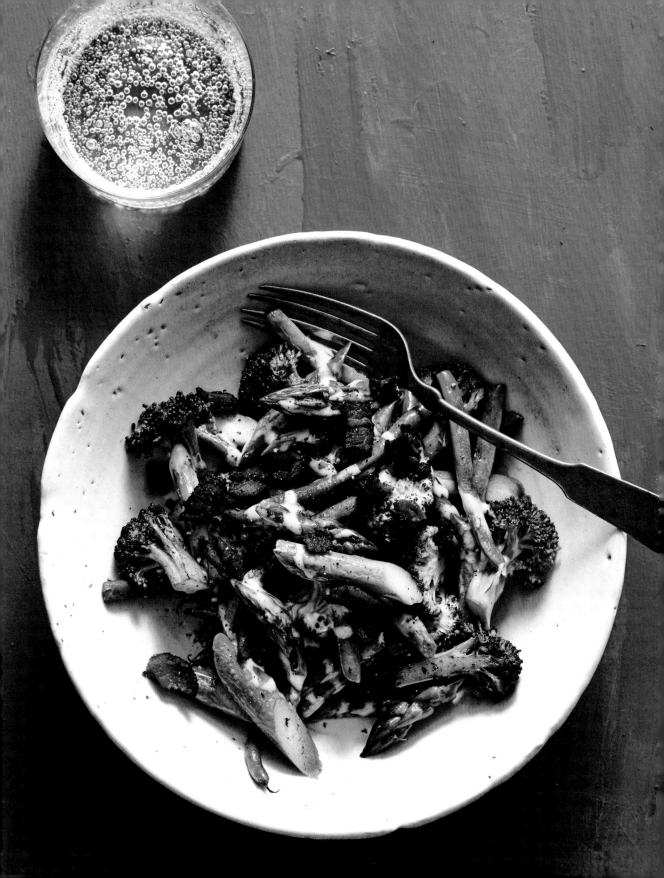

BAKED EGG NOODLE NESTS

These are a riff on eggs and hash browns rolled into one. If you dash out the door in the morning, you can make these ahead of time and reheat them in the morning.

SERVES 3

- 2 tablespoons avocado oil (or avocado oil spray + 1 tablespoon avocado oil)
- 1 pound daikon radish, turnips, or kohlrabi, peeled and cut into noodles (see Tip)
- ½ teaspoon kosher salt
- ¼ teaspoon ground black pepper
- 6 large eggs

MACRONUTRIENTS PER SERVING

CALORIES: 263

FAT: 20 G/180 CALORIES

CARBOHYDRATE: 7 G/ 28 CALORIES

PROTEIN: 13 G/52 CALORIES

1. Preheat the oven to 425°F. Grease 6 cups of a standard muffin tin or silicone muffin cups with 1 tablespoon of the avocado oil (or use avocado oil spray).

2. Divide the vegetable noodles evenly among the 6 cups and press into the bottom. Drizzle each portion with ½ teaspoon avocado oil. Season the noodles with ¼ teaspoon of the salt and ⅛ teaspoon of the pepper. Place them in the oven to bake for 15 minutes.

3. Remove the muffin tin from the oven. Crack 1 egg into each cup on top of the noodles. (Alternatively, you can lightly beat the eggs in a bowl and pour the beaten eggs evenly over the noodles.) Sprinkle with the remaining ¼ teaspoon salt and ⅛ teaspoon pepper. Return the muffin tin to the oven to bake until the eggs are cooked to your liking, 10 to 15 minutes. Remove from the oven and use a large spoon to carefully remove the "nests" from the cups. Serve warm.

TIP: The best tool for this job is a spiralizer. If you don't have one, you can also finely julienne the vegetables or even shred them.

CHOCOLATE PECAN MUFFIN TOPS (EGG-FREE)

This is a great recipe to make with kids. If you do any kind of keto baking, ground flaxseed and psyllium husks should be pantry staples to improve texture of the final product.

SERVES 8

- 2   small zucchini, shredded (about 2 cups)
- ½   cup water
- ½   cup full-fat coconut milk
- 1   teaspoon vanilla extract
- 4   teaspoons ground flaxseeds
- 2   teaspoons ground psyllium husks
- ¼   cup + 2 tablespoons coconut flour, sifted
- 1   teaspoon baking powder, homemade (page 253) or store-bought
- ½   teaspoon ground cinnamon
- ¼   teaspoon sea salt
- ½   teaspoon apple cider vinegar
- 2   scoops (42 g) chocolate-flavored whey protein powder
- 2   teaspoon unsweetened cocoa powder
- ½   cup chopped pecans

1. Preheat the oven to 350°F. Line a baking sheet with parchment paper.

2. Place the shredded zucchini on a clean kitchen towel to drain out some of the liquid.

3. In a medium bowl, combine the water, coconut milk, and vanilla. Stir in the flaxseeds, psyllium husks, coconut flour, baking powder, cinnamon, and salt. Allow this mixture to sit for 10 minutes. The batter will appear very dry.

4. Stir in the vinegar, protein powder, cocoa powder, and pecans and stir well to incorporate. Squeeze the zucchini in the towel to remove additional moisture, then stir it in.

5. Divide the mixture into 8 equal portions. Use your hands to roll each portion into a ball, flatten it slightly, and place it on the parchment paper. Bake until the outside appears dry and it has a bit of resistance when you push on the middle (the middle will remain a bit moist), 45 to 50 minutes. Remove them from the oven and let them sit for 5 minutes before serving.

MACRONUTRIENTS PER SERVING*
CALORIES: 127
FAT: 9 G/82 CALORIES
CARBOHYDRATE: 8 G/ 33 CALORIES
PROTEIN: 5 G/20 CALORIES

* Macros based on using Primal Fuel Chocolate Coconut Protein Powder.

KETO HOME FRIES WITH GREENS

If you miss breakfast potatoes, check out this keto version of home fries. Daikon radish and turnips both make excellent substitutes for potatoes in a low-carb diet. The kale in this recipe isn't generally a component of home fries, but it adds interesting texture (as always with kale) and it's a creative way to get more greens.

SERVES 4

½   bunch (about 4 leaves) curly kale, ends trimmed, central ribs and leaves separated

2   tablespoons + 4 teaspoons butter or ghee

1   daikon radish, peeled and cut into ½-inch cubes

3   small turnips (about 10 ounces), peeled and cut into ½-inch cubes

½   small onion, diced

1   small green bell pepper, diced

1   clove garlic, minced

½   teaspoon kosher salt

½   teaspoon ground black pepper

¼   cup fresh parsley leaves, finely chopped

FOR SERVING (OPTIONAL)

1   tablespoon butter or ghee

4   large eggs

1. Dice the kale ribs and cut the leaves into bite-size pieces, but keep them separate.

2. In a large skillet, melt 2 tablespoons of the butter over medium heat. Add the daikon, reduce the heat a bit, and cook for 5 minutes, stirring frequently.

3. Add the turnips, diced kale ribs, onion, bell pepper, and garlic. Season with the salt and pepper. Cover the pan and cook for 10 minutes, stirring occasionally.

4. Uncover, stir in the kale leaves, and cook a few minutes, until they are tender.

5. Remove from the heat and stir in the parsley. Divide the vegetables among four serving bowls and top each with 1 teaspoon of butter.

6. For the optional topping: In the same skillet, melt the butter and fry the eggs until the yolks are set to your desired doneness. Top each bowl with a fried egg.

7. Serve hot or warm.

Mix it up!
- Chop up cooked sugar-free sausage or bacon and add it to the skillet with the kale leaves in step 4.
- After stirring in the parsley (step 5), sprinkle about 1 cup shredded cheese over all the vegetables and place the lid back on the skillet; let it sit for a few minutes to melt the cheese.

MACRONUTRIENTS PER SERVING (NO EGG)
CALORIES: 172
FAT: 14 G/126 CALORIES
CARBOHYDRATE: 12 G/ 46 CALORIES
PROTEIN: 2 G/8 CALORIES

MACRONUTRIENTS PER SERVING (WITH EGG)
CALORIES: 250
FAT: 19 G/175 CALORIES
CARBOHYDRATE: 12 G/ 48 CALORIES
PROTEIN: 8 G/34 CALORIES

SAVORY SHRIMP MUFFINS

For this recipe, it is often quickest and most economical to use frozen, wild-caught shrimp. You can find them in 1- or 2-pound bags. Thaw what you need for this recipe overnight in the refrigerator, and keep the rest frozen to use later in Keto Shrimp Fried Rice (page 115) or Parmesan Popcorn Shrimp (page 157).

MAKES 6 MUFFINS

Avocado oil spray, or 1 tablespoon coconut oil, melted

1 tablespoon butter or ghee

2 cloves garlic, minced

16 small shrimp, peeled, deveined, and tails removed

1 teaspoon kosher salt

½ teaspoon ground black pepper

1 medium zucchini, grated (about 1 packed cup)

2 large eggs

2 tablespoons coconut flour

¼ teaspoon baking soda

2 teaspoons fresh lime juice

2 tablespoons fresh cilantro leaves, finely chopped

MACRONUTRIENTS PER MUFFIN

CALORIES: 92

FAT: 7 G/63 CALORIES

CARBOHYDRATE: 3 G/ 12 CALORIES

PROTEIN: 5 G/20 CALORIES

1. Preheat the oven to 350°F. Grease 6 cups of a standard muffin tin—or, even better, silicone muffin cups—with the avocado oil spray or coconut oil.

2. In a medium skillet, melt the butter over medium heat. Add the garlic and sauté for 30 seconds. Add the shrimp and season with ¼ teaspoon each of the salt and pepper. Sauté until the shrimp are just opaque, 1 to 2 minutes. Remove the skillet from the heat. Use tongs to transfer the shrimp to a cutting board. Hold on to the skillet with the garlic in it.

3. Place the zucchini in a clean kitchen towel and roll it up. Press down firmly on the towel to squeeze out excess water.

4. In a medium bowl, lightly beat the eggs with the remaining ¾ teaspoon salt and ¼ teaspoon pepper. Sift in the coconut flour and baking soda and stir well. Add the grated zucchini, lime juice, and cilantro. Use a spatula to scrape the butter and garlic out of the skillet into the batter. Stir well again.

5. Roughly chop the shrimp. Stir it into the batter.

6. Divide the batter evenly among the muffin cups. Bake until a toothpick inserted into the middle comes out clean, 25 to 30 minutes. Remove the muffins from the oven and let sit for 5 minutes to cool. Serve warm.

SMOKED SALMON STACKS

The flavors in this recipe are a classic combo, but you would normally expect to find them served on a bagel. You can assemble these the night before and grab them on your way out the door in the morning. They also make a great lunchbox option for adventurous primal kids.

SERVES 2

3 tablespoons full-fat cream cheese, at room temperature

3 tablespoons goat cheese

2 tablespoons capers, drained

2 teaspoons chopped fresh chives (optional)

1 cucumber, cut into 16 thin slices

¼ red onion, sliced as thinly as possible (or substitute pickled red onion)

3 small Roma (plum) tomatoes, cut into 16 thin slices

4 ounces smoked salmon, divided into 16 portions

MACRONUTRIENTS PER SERVING (8 STACKS)

CALORIES: 279

FAT: 17 G/153 CALORIES

CARBOHYDRATE: 12 G/ 48 CALORIES

PROTEIN: 20 G/80 CALORIES

1. In a small bowl, combine the cream cheese, goat cheese, capers, and chives (if using). Mix with a fork until well incorporated. This can be done the day before to save time.

2. Assemble the stacks by spreading about 1 teaspoon of the cheese mixture on each slice of cucumber. Press a small portion of the sliced red onion into the cheese mixture. Top with a slice of tomato and a piece of smoked salmon. If necessary, secure each stack with a toothpick.

3. Serve immediately, or store in an airtight container in the refrigerator until ready to serve.

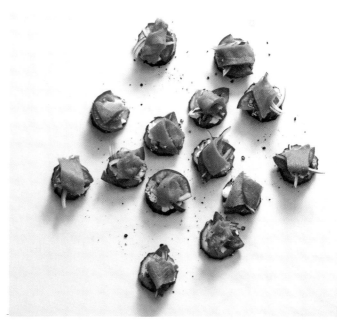

SOUPS & SALADS

BROCCOLI-CAULIFLOWER SOUP

Sure, you can make cauliflower soup *or* broccoli soup, but have you ever made cauliflower *and* broccoli soup?? This recipe is written to be dairy-free, but if cheesy soup is what you're after, see the Note.

SERVES 6

2	tablespoons coconut oil
½	medium onion, chopped
1	large stalk celery, chopped
3 to 4	kale ribs, chopped (optional)
1	clove garlic, minced
3	cups broccoli florets
3	cups cauliflower florets
4	cups chicken bone broth (page 35) or vegetable stock
	Sea salt
½	teaspoon ground black pepper
½	teaspoon ground nutmeg
1	cup full-fat coconut milk (see Note)

1. In a large pot, heat the coconut oil over medium heat. Add the onion, celery, and kale ribs (if using) and sauté until the vegetables are soft, about 5 minutes. Add the garlic and sauté 1 minute more.

2. Stir in the broccoli, cauliflower, broth, 1 teaspoon salt, the pepper, and nutmeg. Bring the soup to a boil, then reduce the heat to a simmer and cook, stirring occasionally, until the broccoli and cauliflower are very soft and easily pierced with a fork, about 20 minutes.

3. Use an immersion blender to blend the soup until smooth. (Alternatively, working in batches, *carefully* transfer the soup to a regular blender and blend it until smooth. Do not overfill the blender.)

4. Add the coconut milk to the soup and stir to combine. Taste and adjust the salt. Ladle it into individual serving bowls.

Note: If you are not dairy-free, you can substitute heavy whipping cream for the coconut milk. As long as you're at it, why not throw in a big handful of shredded cheese (cheddar or Gruyère are both great options) after you blend the soup? Feta cheese also goes quite nicely with this soup.

MACRONUTRIENTS PER SERVING

CALORIES: 183

FAT: 14 G/130 CALORIES

CARBOHYDRATE: 9 G/ 36 CALORIES

PROTEIN: 7 G/26 CALORIES

HAM SALAD

This salad gives off major 1950s throwback vibes (without all the Jell-O). It's a great way to use up leftover holiday ham. Serve it over a bed of greens or in lettuce cups.

SERVES 2

- ¼ cup avocado oil mayonnaise
- 2 teaspoons Dijon mustard
- ¼ teaspoon dried dill
- ¼ teaspoon ground black pepper

  Dash of cayenne pepper (optional)

- 1 cup (about 8 ounces) diced cooked ham (see Note)
- 1 stalk celery, finely chopped
- 2 tablespoons finely chopped dill pickle

In a small bowl, mix the mayo, mustard, dill, black pepper, and cayenne (if using). Stir in the ham, celery, and dill pickle. Serve immediately, or transfer to an airtight container and store in the refrigerator for up to 3 days.

Note: If you intend to eat this by itself or on top of a green leafy salad, cut the ham into about ½-inch cubes. However, you can also dice it smaller or even use a food processor to grind it up if you want a more uniform texture.

Mix it up! Try adding chopped green olives, pimientos, or shredded cheddar cheese. You can also add chopped hard-boiled eggs; if so, you might want to add another 2 teaspoons or so of mayo for each egg.

MACRONUTRIENTS PER SERVING
CALORIES: 390
FAT: 29 G/264 CALORIES
CARBOHYDRATE: 4 G/16 CALORIES
PROTEIN: 26 G/104 CALORIES

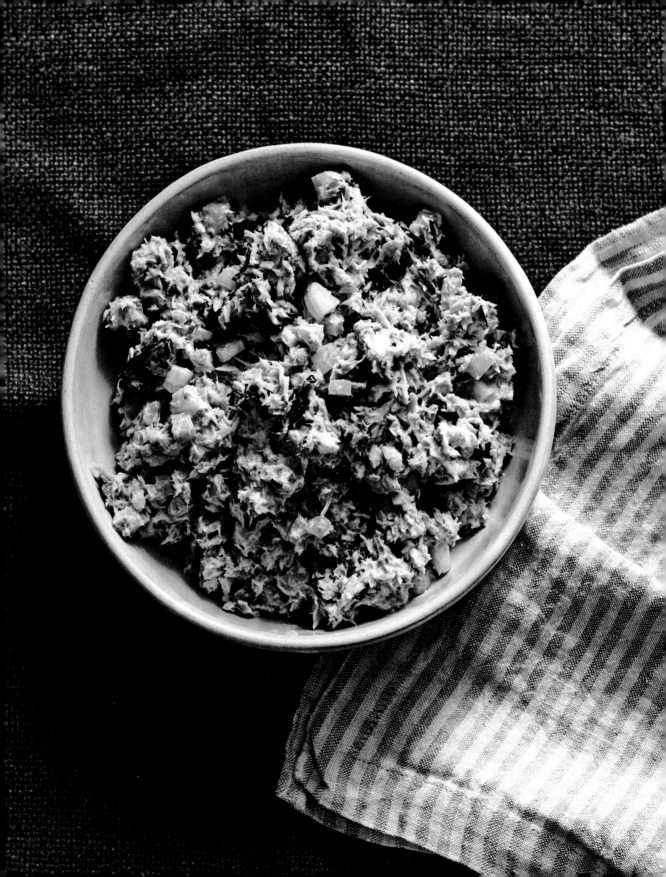

THREE FROM THE SEA SALAD

This is not your average tuna salad! This unique preparation is a gateway to enjoying more of the awesome omega-3 benefits of sardines for those who aren't so excited to eat them alone. Dulse is a type of seaweed whose flavor is reminiscent of bacon, believe it or not. It is quite chewy when it is dry, but once it sits in the salad for a few minutes it softens right up. Look for dulse with nori and other dried seaweed in the Asian foods section of your grocery store or online. Be sure to choose products that are free of added vegetable oils, which unfortunately are often found in seaweed products.

SERVES 2

1   (5-ounce) can albacore tuna (see Note)

1   (4.4-ounce) can sardines packed in olive oil

1   stalk celery, diced

¼   cup dried dulse

2   tablespoons avocado oil mayonnaise

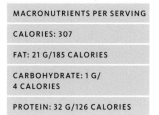

MACRONUTRIENTS PER SERVING
CALORIES: 307
FAT: 21 G/185 CALORIES
CARBOHYDRATE: 1 G/ 4 CALORIES
PROTEIN: 32 G/126 CALORIES

1. In a small bowl, combine the tuna, sardines, and the oil from both cans. Use a fork to break up the fish into small pieces and mix them together. Stir in the diced celery.

2. Use a sharp knife or kitchen shears to roughly chop the dulse. Dried dulse can be a bit tough, so do not worry about chopping it too fine. Add it to the bowl.

3. Add the mayo and stir thoroughly to combine. Serve immediately, or let it sit for a few minutes to soften the dulse.

Note: High-quality canned albacore tuna, like Wild Planet and Safe Catch brands, will only have tuna and salt listed as ingredients. The oil in the can is from the fish itself. Strictly avoid tuna packed in vegetable oil or sunflower oil.

SUPER GREENS EGG DROP SOUP

Here's another great way to add greens to a dish that wouldn't traditionally have them. The pleasant bitterness of the dandelion leaves contrasts with the mild sweetness of the baby bok choy in a most pleasing way here.

SERVES 6

2 cups loosely packed dandelion leaves (see Notes), chopped small

2 cups loosely packed baby spinach, chopped small

2 small baby bok choy (4 ounces total), cores removed, leaves chopped small

4 scallions, chopped

1 large clove garlic, minced

2 teaspoons finely minced fresh ginger

2 tablespoons tamari or coconut aminos

4 cups chicken bone broth, preferably homemade (page 35)

2 cups filtered water

Sea salt

3 large eggs

Juice of 1/3 to 1/2 lemon, to taste

About 1 tablespoon kelp flakes (optional; see Notes)

1. In a large stockpot, combine the dandelion, spinach, bok choy, scallions, garlic, ginger, tamari, broth, water, and 1/2 teaspoon salt. Bring the mixture to a boil, then reduce to a simmer and simmer until the greens are very tender, about 15 minutes. Taste and adjust the salt.

2. Crack the eggs into a bowl and beat them lightly with a fork. Stir the soup in a circular motion to get the soup swirling in the pot. Slowly stream the egg into the hot soup. The eggs will cook in the soup, forming ribbons.

3. Stir in the lemon juice. Taste and adjust the salt again. Ladle the vegetables and broth into serving bowls, sprinkle with kelp flakes (if using), and serve hot.

Notes
- If you can't find dandelion leaves in your market, simply substitute additional baby bok choy.
- Kelp is the best dietary source of iodine, a nutrient that is essential for proper thyroid function. Look for kelp flakes with the spices in your grocery store. They come in a container that looks like a salt shaker.

MACRONUTRIENTS PER SERVING
CALORIES: 122
FAT: 5 G/44 CALORIES
CARBOHYDRATE: 11 G/ 44 CALORIES
PROTEIN: 9 G/36 CALORIES

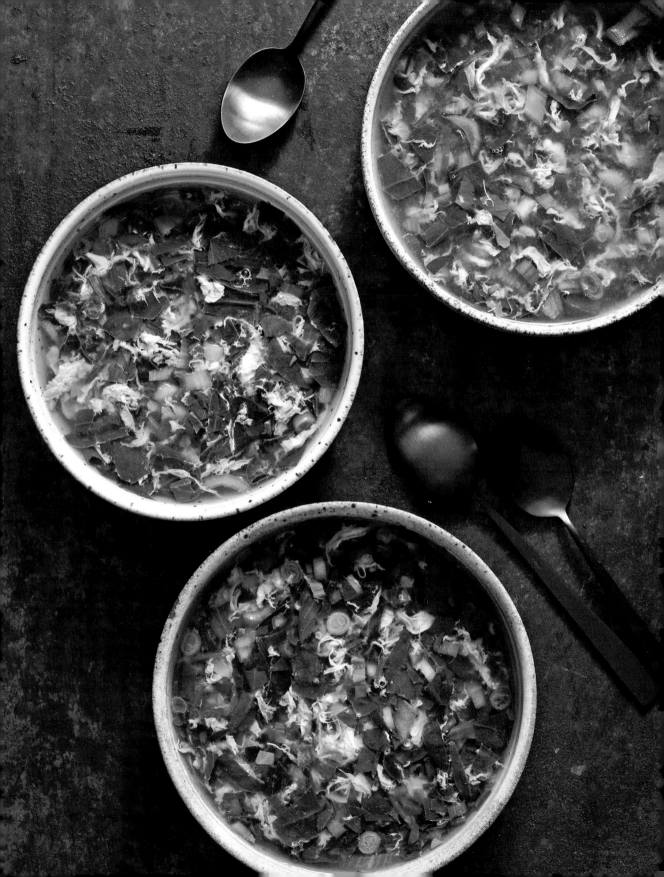

GRILLED ROMAINE SALAD WITH ANCHOVIES

Anchovies are unfairly maligned thanks to their reputation as the world's worst pizza topping. But us primal and keto folks know that oily, cold-water fish from the SMASH hits list (sardines, mackerel, anchovies, salmon, herring) are true superfoods with more nutrient density than any other fish. Add grilled or rotisserie chicken for a complete meal.

SERVES 4

FOR THE DRESSING

- 2   teaspoons Dijon mustard
- 2   cloves garlic, chopped
- 1   (1.6-ounce) tin anchovy fillets packed in olive oil
- 2   tablespoons fresh lemon juice
- 2   tablespoons apple cider vinegar
- ½   cup extra-virgin olive oil
      Sea salt (optional)

FOR THE SALAD

- 2   small heads romaine lettuce
- 1   tablespoon avocado oil
- ½   lemon
- ½   teaspoon sea salt
- ½   teaspoon ground black pepper
- ½   cup shredded Parmesan cheese (optional)
- 1   (1.6-ounce) tin anchovy fillets packed in olive oil

1. For the dressing: In a high-powered blender (see Note), combine the mustard, garlic, anchovies, the oil from the tin, the lemon juice, and vinegar. Blend for 15 to 20 seconds to combine the ingredients. With the blender running, slowly stream in the olive oil. Once all the olive oil is added, continue blending for another 5 to 10 seconds. Taste and add salt if desired.

2. Heat an outdoor grill or indoor grill pan over medium-high heat.

3. For the salad: Remove any loose or damaged exterior leaves from the romaine (save any loose leaves for burger or lunch meat wraps). Use a sharp knife to halve each head of romaine lengthwise, directly through the core. Brush the cut sides with the avocado oil, squeeze the lemon juice over them, and season with salt and pepper.

4. Place the romaine cut side down on the hot grill. Grill until it is just starting to char, 3 to 5 minutes. Carefully flip the romaine and sprinkle with the Parmesan (if using). Grill another 3 minutes. Remove to a serving platter.

5. Top the romaine with the anchovies and drizzle with the dressing. Serve warm or at room temperature.

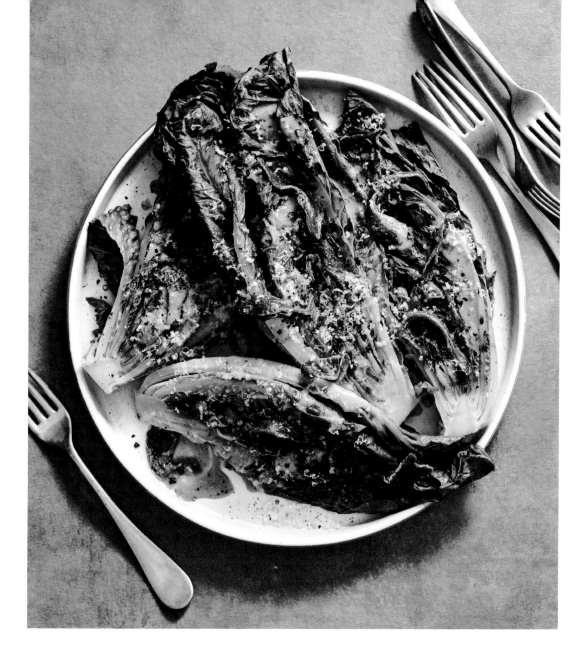

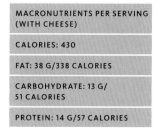

MACRONUTRIENTS PER SERVING (WITH CHEESE)
CALORIES: 430
FAT: 38 G/338 CALORIES
CARBOHYDRATE: 13 G/ 51 CALORIES
PROTEIN: 14 G/57 CALORIES

Note: The dressing can also be made with an immersion blender in a jar that tightly fits the blender. This dressing is essentially a Caesar dressing without the egg and cheese. If you want to make it a more traditional Caesar dressing, add one room-temperature egg yolk in the initial step. After streaming in the olive oil, add ¼ cup shredded Parmesan cheese and pulse a few times to combine.

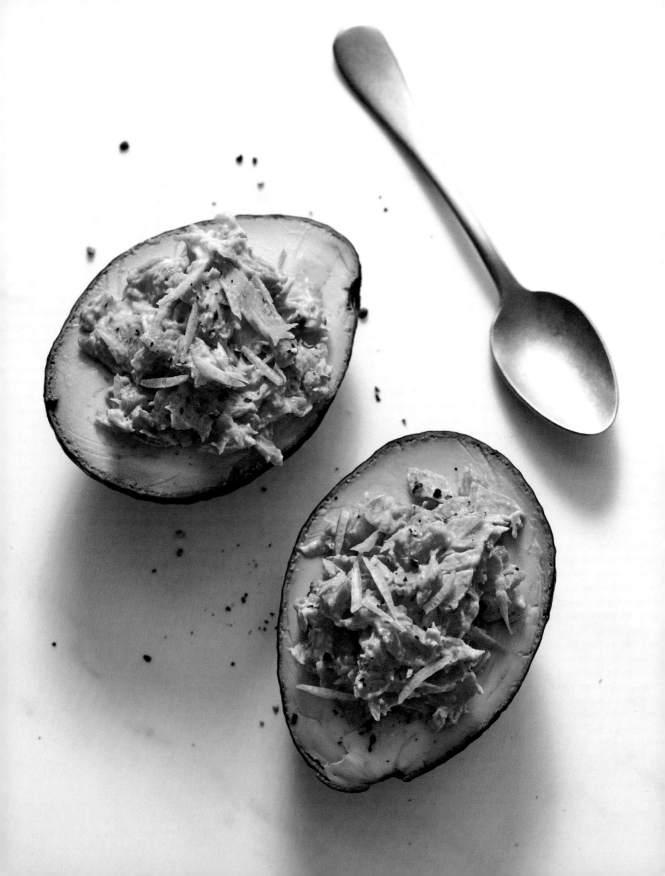

AVOCADO STUFFED WITH SALMON SALAD

Serve this dish over a bed of greens with a side of grilled vegetables for a light and easy meal.

- 2 ounces cooked salmon (leftover or canned)
- 2 ounces smoked salmon, finely chopped
- 2 tablespoons avocado oil mayonnaise
- ½ teaspoon grated lemon zest
- ¾ teaspoon fresh lemon juice
- ⅛ teaspoon celery salt or sea salt
- ⅛ teaspoon ground black pepper
- 1 avocado

MACRONUTRIENTS PER SIDE SERVING (½ RECIPE)

CALORIES: 300

FAT: 25 G/225 CALORIES

CARBOHYDRATE: 7 G/ 26 CALORIES

PROTEIN: 14 G/55 CALORIES

1. Flake the cooked salmon into a medium bowl. Add the smoked salmon, mayo, lemon zest, lemon juice, celery salt, and pepper and stir very well to combine. At this point you can refrigerate the salmon salad until ready to eat.

2. When you are ready to serve, halve the avocado lengthwise and carefully remove the pit. Scoop a little bit of the flesh of the avocado out to make a "bowl" to hold the filling. Place the scooped out avocado in a small bowl and mash it with a fork. Add the mashed avocado to the salmon mix and stir to combine.

3. Place the avocado "bowls" on a plate. If they are rolling to one side, you can carefully cut a piece off the bottom with a very sharp knife to create a flat base. Divide the salmon mixture evenly between the two halves of the avocado, gently packing it into the divots and mounding it on top. Serve immediately.

SHREDDED TABBOULEH SALAD

This salad invokes the flavors of tabbouleh (a.k.a. tabouli or tabbouli) without relying on the grains that are usually the basis of a tabbouleh salad. If you eat dairy, crumbled feta or goat cheese is a tasty addition to this recipe.

SERVES 4

4   cups finely shredded green cabbage (about 8 ounces)

16   grape tomatoes, halved

1   small cucumber, peeled and diced

3   scallions, chopped

3   tablespoons finely chopped fresh flat-leaf parsley

1   tablespoon finely chopped fresh mint

3   tablespoons extra-virgin olive oil

1   tablespoon fresh lemon juice

1   teaspoon minced garlic

½   teaspoon sea salt

½   teaspoon ground black pepper

MACRONUTRIENTS PER SERVING

CALORIES: 129

FAT: 10 G/94 CALORIES

CARBOHYDRATE: 9 G/ 36 CALORIES

PROTEIN: 2 G/8 CALORIES

In a large bowl, combine the cabbage, tomatoes, cucumber, scallions, herbs, oil, lemon juice, garlic, salt, and pepper and stir very well. Taste and adjust the salt and pepper. Place in the refrigerator to rest for at least 1 hour before serving, or overnight.

Mix it up! Replace the green cabbage with shredded raw Brussels sprouts or massaged kale (see Kale Salad with Pumpkin "Croutons" on page 92 for how to massage kale).

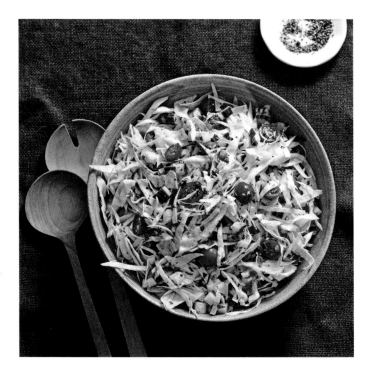

BLUEBERRIES AND FETA SALAD

This simple recipe is a hit thanks to the way the sweetness of the blueberries is offset by the sharpness of the feta cheese. Look for fresh feta packed in brine for maximum tangy flavor.

SERVES 2 AS A
SIDE SALAD

4   cups packed dark leafy salad greens (arugula, baby spinach, baby kale, etc.)

4   tablespoons balsamic vinaigrette dressing, or dressing of choice

½   cup broccoli sprouts or other microgreens (optional)

⅓   cup blueberries

¼   cup crumbled feta cheese

     Ground black pepper (optional)

1. Toss the salad greens with 2 tablespoons of the salad dressing and divide the greens between two plates or salad bowls. Sprinkle the sprouts or microgreens over the top if desired.

2. Divide the blueberries and feta cheese between the salads. If desired, crack a bit of black pepper over the top. Drizzle with the remaining 2 tablespoons dressing. Serve immediately.

MACRONUTRIENTS PER SERVING*

CALORIES: 210

FAT: 18 G/159 CALORIES

CARBOHYDRATE: 10 G/ 40 CALORIES

PROTEIN: 6 G/25 CALORIES

* Macros based on using Primal Kitchen Balsamic Vinaigrette.

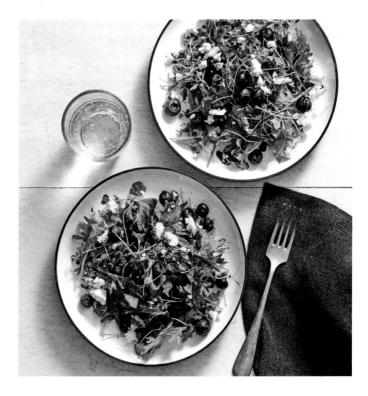

AVGOLEMONO (LEMON CHICKEN SOUP)

This traditional Greek soup is perfect for a keto diet . . . except for the orzo or rice with which it is traditionally made. No worries, an easy swap with keto superstar cauliflower rice, and we're back in business!

SERVES 6

1 tablespoon avocado oil

2 stalks celery, chopped

½ cup chopped onion

2 cloves garlic, chopped

8 cups chicken bone broth, preferably homemade (page 35)

2 cups filtered water

2 bay leaves

2 cups diced cooked chicken

2 cups riced cauliflower (fresh or thawed frozen)

3 large eggs

½ cup fresh lemon juice

3 tablespoons butter or ghee, melted

Sea salt and ground black pepper

MACRONUTRIENTS PER SERVING

CALORIES: 305

FAT: 17 G/151 CALORIES

CARBOHYDRATE: 6 G/ 25 CALORIES

PROTEIN: 32 G/126 CALORIES

1. In a large pot, heat the avocado oil over medium-high heat. Add the celery and onion and sauté, stirring frequently, until the vegetables are soft, about 3 minutes. Stir in the garlic and sauté another 30 seconds.

2. Carefully pour the broth and water into the pot and add the bay leaves. Bring the liquid to a boil, then reduce the heat to a simmer and simmer for 20 minutes to meld the flavors.

3. Ladle about 1 cup of the broth into a measuring cup with a pouring spout. Set aside. Add the cooked chicken and the riced cauliflower to the pot and stir.

4. In a medium bowl, lightly beat the eggs. Lightly beat in the lemon juice. Slowly pour in a few tablespoons of the reserved hot broth from the measuring cup, whisking the whole time. Continue to whisk the reserved broth into the eggs until the entire cup of broth has been incorporated. Whisk in the melted butter until completely combined.

5. Slowly pour the egg mixture back into the soup pot, stirring constantly. Check the consistency of the cauliflower rice. It should be tender. If not, continue to simmer until the cauliflower is the right consistency. Taste and season with salt and pepper. Remove the bay leaves and serve immediately.

FENNEL SALAD WITH AVOCADO GREEN GODDESS DRESSING

When set against a creamy avocado dressing, the flavors and crunchiness of raw fennel and kohlrabi really shine. For a little extra hit of the licorice-y flavor fennel offers, reserve a few fronds, finely chop them, and sprinkle them over the finished salad.

SERVES 4

FOR THE DRESSING

- ½ avocado
- ½ cup avocado oil mayonnaise
- About ½ cup loosely packed fresh herbs (see Note), leaves only
- 1 clove garlic, chopped
- 1 tablespoon fresh lemon juice (preferably Meyer lemon)
- Scant ¼ teaspoon ground black pepper
- Filtered water

FOR THE SALAD

- 1 cup thinly sliced fennel
- 1 cup peeled kohlrabi, julienned
- 2 teaspoons fresh lemon juice (preferably Meyer lemon)
- ¼ teaspoon sea salt
- 8 cups dark leafy greens, such as spinach, chard, baby kale, or a mix
- ¼ cup sunflower seeds

1. For the dressing: In a blender, combine the avocado, mayo, herbs, garlic, lemon juice, and pepper and blend until smooth. With the blender running on low, add water 1 tablespoon at a time until the dressing reaches the desired consistency. Set aside.

2. For the salad: In a small bowl, toss the sliced fennel and kohlrabi with the lemon juice and salt. In a large bowl, toss the fennel and kohlrabi with the greens. Divide the salads among four small bowls. Top with a generous dollop of dressing and sprinkle with sunflower seeds. Serve immediately.

Note: Recommended herb blend: ¼ cup parsley, 3 tablespoons cilantro, and 2 teaspoons chives. You can also add fresh mint, tarragon, or basil.

MACRONUTRIENTS PER SERVING
CALORIES: 316
FAT: 29 G/264 CALORIES
CARBOHYDRATE: 12 G/ 48 CALORIES
PROTEIN: 5 G/21 CALORIES

TURKEY TURMERIC SOUP

There are a lot of flavors happening in this soup, but it all works. The fresh and the dried turmeric each lend their own flavor, so include both if you can.

SERVES 4

- 2 tablespoons ghee or fat of choice
- 1 small bunch kale (about 6 leaves), preferably lacinato, ribs and leaves separated
- 1 small onion, finely chopped
- 1 tablespoon finely grated fresh ginger
- 6 cloves garlic, finely chopped

  2-inch piece fresh turmeric root, peeled and finely grated
- ¾ teaspoon ground turmeric
- 1 pound ground turkey (thigh or breast)
- ½ teaspoon ground coriander
- ¼ teaspoon ground cinnamon

  Kosher salt and ground black pepper
- ¼ teaspoon cayenne pepper (optional)
- ¼ cup chopped fresh cilantro
- 6 cups chicken bone broth, homemade (page 35) or store-bought

  Juice of ½ lemon

1. In a large soup pot, heat the ghee over medium heat. Dice the kale ribs.

2. When the ghee is hot, add the kale ribs and onion and sauté until they start to soften, about 4 minutes. Add the ginger and garlic and sauté, stirring constantly, for 2 minutes more.

3. Add the fresh and ground turmeric and sauté 1 minute more, stirring constantly.

4. Use your hands to crumble in the ground turkey. Sprinkle in the coriander, cinnamon, 1 teaspoon salt, ¼ teaspoon black pepper, the cayenne (if using), and the fresh cilantro. Stir very well. Cook until the turkey is just cooked through, 5 to 7 minutes, breaking up the meat as it cooks.

5. Pour in about ½ cup broth and deglaze the pan, using a wooden spoon to scrape up any browned bits. Add the rest of the broth and bring to a boil, reduce the heat to medium-low, and simmer for 10 minutes, stirring occasionally.

6. Chop the kale leaves into small pieces. Add them to the soup and simmer another few minutes until the kale leaves are soft. Taste and adjust the salt and black pepper. Stir in the lemon juice just before serving.

MACRONUTRIENTS PER SERVING

CALORIES: 372

FAT: 26 G/234 CALORIES

CARBOHYDRATE: 7 G/ 28 CALORIES

PROTEIN: 30 G/120 CALORIES

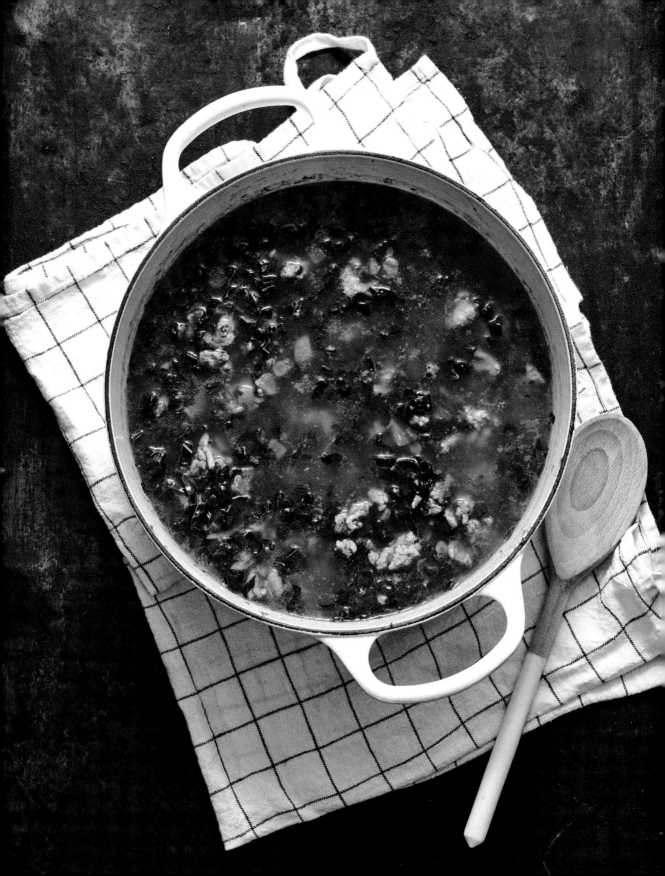

CUCUMBER YOGURT SALAD

This salad is even better after it sits for a few hours, so go ahead and make it ahead of time. The recipe can easily be doubled or more for bringing to a potluck or picnic.

SERVES 4

1   large English cucumber

¼   cup plain full-fat kefir (dairy or coconut milk; see Note)

1   clove garlic, pressed or very finely minced

¼   cup fresh parsley leaves, very finely chopped

1   teaspoon finely chopped fresh dill

½   teaspoon grated lemon zest

1   teaspoon fresh lemon juice

     Kosher salt

⅛   teaspoon ground black pepper

1. Stripe the cucumber by lightly peeling it but leaving some green. Quarter the cucumber lengthwise and remove the seeds with a spoon. Cut the cucumber crosswise into ¼-inch-thick pieces.

2. In a medium bowl, combine the kefir, garlic, parsley, dill, lemon zest, lemon juice, ¼ teaspoon salt, and the pepper. Taste and adjust the salt. Gently stir in the cucumber slices.

3. Cover the cucumber salad and refrigerate for at least 1 hour but up to overnight. Before serving, stir well.

Note: You can substitute plain full-fat Greek yogurt thinned out with a bit of water to approximate kefir.

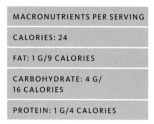

MACRONUTRIENTS PER SERVING

CALORIES: 24

FAT: 1 G/9 CALORIES

CARBOHYDRATE: 4 G/ 16 CALORIES

PROTEIN: 1 G/4 CALORIES

DILL PICKLE SOUP

In our Keto Reset Facebook community, new members sometimes ask how to deal with cravings for sweets. Dill pickles can do the trick! Something about the crunchiness and the salty acidity of the brined pickles knocks down cravings without feeding the sugar monster.

SERVES 4

2 tablespoons ghee or fat of choice

1 small onion, diced

3 stalks celery with leaves, diced

5 cups stock (vegetable or chicken)

1 small head cauliflower, cut into florets and roughly chopped

1 cup daikon radish, peeled and sliced

4 tablespoons unsalted butter, melted (or additional ghee)

1 large egg (optional)

3 large dill pickles, finely diced (about ¾ cup), plus 8 slices dill pickle, for garnish (optional)

½ cup pickle juice/brine

½ teaspoon ground black pepper

Sea salt

Keto-friendly hot sauce to taste (optional)

1. In a large stockpot, heat the ghee over medium heat. Add the onion and celery and sauté until the vegetables are soft, about 5 minutes. Add the stock, cauliflower, and daikon. Bring to a boil, then reduce the heat, cover, and simmer until the vegetables are soft, about 15 minutes.

2. Add the melted butter to the soup. Use a potato masher or immersion blender to break up the vegetables and incorporate them into the soup, leaving some chunkiness.

3. For a thicker soup: Ladle about 1 cup of the broth into a small measuring cup with a pouring spout. Crack the egg into a bowl and beat it lightly. Very slowly pour the hot broth into the egg, whisking the whole time. Slowly pour the egg mixture back into the soup, stirring vigorously the whole time.

4. Stir the diced pickles and the pickle juice into the soup, along with the pepper. Simmer for 10 minutes more to allow the flavors to meld. Taste and add more pepper and additional salt if desired.

5. Ladle the soup into individual bowls. If desired, top each bowl with a dash of hot sauce and 2 slices of dill pickle.

MACRONUTRIENTS PER SERVING (WITH EGG)
CALORIES: 291
FAT: 24 G/212 CALORIES
CARBOHYDRATE: 11 G/ 45 CALORIES
PROTEIN: 11 G/43 CALORIES

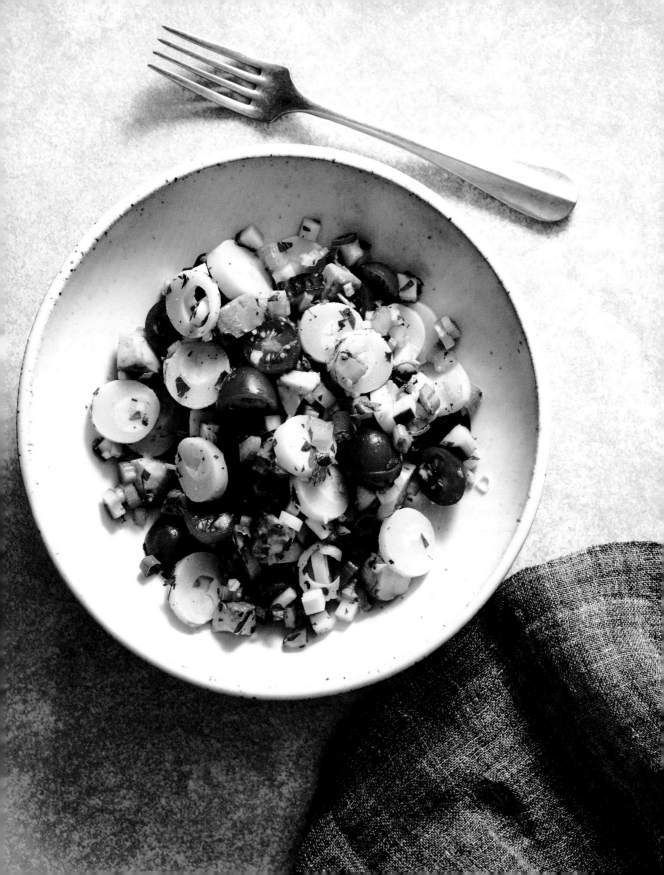

HEARTS OF PALM SALAD

If you have never tried hearts of palm—the edible core of certain palm trees—this Brazilian-inspired salad is a great introduction. Hearts of palm have a mild flavor, akin to bamboo shoots, that pairs beautifully with baked fish, grilled shrimp, or even a juicy steak.

SERVES 4

FOR THE DRESSING

- 3 tablespoons extra-virgin olive oil
- 2 tablespoons minced shallots
- 1 clove garlic, pressed or very finely minced
- 1 tablespoon fresh lime juice
- ¼ teaspoon sea salt
- ⅛ teaspoon ground black pepper

FOR THE SALAD

- 1 (14-ounce) can hearts of palm, drained and sliced
- 1 small cucumber, diced
- 12 grape tomatoes, halved
- 2 stalks celery with leaves, finely chopped
- 2 scallions, finely chopped
- ¼ cup loosely packed fresh parsley leaves, chopped
- 1 avocado, cubed

1. For the dressing: In a bowl, whisk together the olive oil, shallots, garlic, lime juice, salt, and pepper.

2. For the salad: In a medium bowl, toss together the hearts of palm, cucumber, tomatoes, celery, scallions, and parsley. Pour the dressing over the salad and toss lightly. Gently stir the avocado into the salad. Serve immediately.

MACRONUTRIENTS PER SERVING

CALORIES: 197

FAT: 16 G/144 CALORIES

CARBOHYDRATE: 13 G/ 52 CALORIES

PROTEIN: 4 G/16 CALORIES

KALE SALAD WITH PUMPKIN "CROUTONS"

If you own *The Keto Reset Diet*, you are probably familiar with the concept of massaging kale. It helps break down the kale, improving both the texture and the flavor. This particular massaged kale salad is perfect for fall. Don't fear the pumpkin "croutons"—pumpkin is a nutrient-dense source of healthy carbs that can be enjoyed in moderation on a keto diet.

SERVES 4

½   cup Homemade Pumpkin Puree (page 245) or unsweetened canned

1   small bunch curly kale (green or red), ribs and leaves separated

1   tablespoon extra-virgin olive oil

1   teaspoon fresh lemon juice

½   teaspoon kosher salt

1   small bunch Swiss chard, ribs and leaves separated

4   tablespoons keto-friendly dressing of choice

¼   teaspoon Pumpkin Pie Spice Blend (page 254)

2   tablespoons coconut oil

½   cup crumbled goat cheese

3   tablespoons pumpkin seeds or sunflower seeds

½   cup raspberries or blackberries (optional)

1. If you are using homemade pumpkin puree, line a sieve with a clean kitchen towel and place it over a bowl. Scoop the pumpkin puree into the towel and set aside. You can skip this step if you are using canned pumpkin, or if your homemade pumpkin is not too watery.

2. Tear or cut the kale leaves into roughly bite-size pieces and place them in a large bowl. Add the olive oil, lemon juice, and ¼ teaspoon of the salt. Use your hands to knead (massage) the kale for about 2 minutes, until the volume has reduced by half.

3. Chop the Swiss chard leaves into small pieces and mix it into the kale. Pour in 2 tablespoons of the dressing and stir well. Set aside.

4. Place the pumpkin in a small bowl. Stir in the pumpkin pie spice and remaining ¼ teaspoon salt. In a skillet, heat the coconut oil over medium heat for 2 minutes. When it is hot, carefully drop rounded teaspoons of the pumpkin mixture into the oil (watch for splatter) and press down to flatten slightly. Work in batches to avoid crowding the pan. Cook until browned on the first side, about 2 minutes. Flip and cook 2 minutes on the second side. Remove the pumpkin

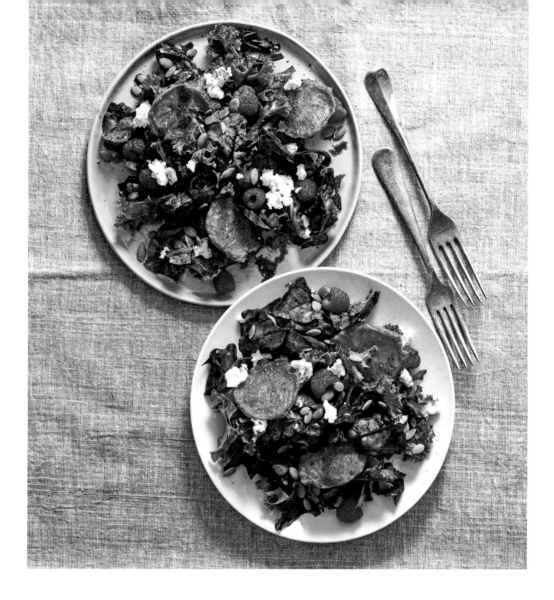

MACRONUTRIENTS PER
SERVING*

CALORIES: 396

FAT: 33 G/297 CALORIES

CARBOHYDRATE: 13 G/
52 CALORIES

PROTEIN: 14 G/56 CALORIES

* Macros based on using Primal Kitchen
Balsamic Vinaigrette.

"croutons" to a plate and repeat until you have used all the
pumpkin mixture. Add more oil if the pan gets too dry.

5. Dice the chard and kale ribs. Add them to the skillet and
stir-fry for about 4 minutes. Mix them into the salad.

6. Transfer the kale and chard mixture to a serving bowl.
Crumble the goat cheese over top, then sprinkle on the
pumpkin seeds. Arrange the berries (if using) and the
pumpkin "croutons" on top. Drizzle with the remaining
2 tablespoons dressing. Serve immediately.

SPICY THAI CHICKEN "NOODLE" SOUP

The aroma that fills your house when you make chicken soup from scratch is one of the coziest things in the world! It takes a little time but the final product is worth it.

SERVES 6

1   whole chicken (about 4 pounds)

1   carrot, sliced

2   stalks celery with leaves, sliced

1   small onion, diced

2   bay leaves
    Kosher salt

8   cups filtered water

1   tablespoon Thai curry paste, panang or red

4   cloves garlic, minced

1   tablespoon minced or microplaned fresh ginger

2   stalks lemongrass, cut in half lengthwise and lightly pounded

MACRONUTRIENTS PER SERVING
CALORIES: 373
FAT: 25 G/224 CALORIES
CARBOHYDRATE: 7 G/ 27 CALORIES
PROTEIN: 31 G/122 CALORIES

1. Place the chicken in a large stockpot along with the carrot, celery, onion, bay leaves, and 1 tablespoon salt. If the neck and gizzards were in the cavity of the chicken, you can add them, too. Add the water, making sure the chicken is covered by at least 1 inch. Bring the water to a boil, then reduce the heat to a simmer. Simmer until the chicken is cooked through, about 1 hour 30 minutes.

2. Carefully remove the chicken and place it in a bowl. Set a large metal sieve over a second large bowl or pot and carefully strain the broth. Discard the solids. Return 5 cups of stock to the soup pot and place it back over low heat.

3. Measure out another 1 cup of stock. In a small bowl, whisk the stock with the curry paste. (Refrigerate or freeze any remaining stock.) Add the curried stock to the soup pot. Stir in the garlic, ginger, lemongrass, and fish sauce. Simmer for 20 minutes.

4. While the soup simmers, cut the zucchini into thin noodles using the smallest blade on your spiralizer or other noodle-cutting tool. Cut the noodles into shorter pieces.

5. When the chicken is cool enough to handle, remove the meat from the bones (see Note). Roughly chop the white and dark meat together, 2 to 3 cups total. (If you have extra meat, place it in an airtight container in the refrigerator.)

6. After the soup has simmered for 20 minutes, remove the lemongrass stalks. Add the chopped chicken to the soup, along with the scallions, coconut milk, and lime juice. Simmer for another 5 minutes. Add the zucchini noodles and simmer just until the noodles are softened, another couple minutes. Taste and adjust the salt.

7. Ladle the soup into bowls. Top each serving with avocado and cilantro (if using). Serve hot.

Note: After you remove the meat from the bones, place the carcass in your slow cooker, along with additional carrots, celery, onion, bay leaf, and some peppercorns. Cover with water and cook on low overnight for more bone broth. Use it to make Golden Bone Broth (page 247) or Garlicky Bone Broth (page 246) tomorrow! Refer to the directions on page 35 for guidance on making your own bone broth.

2	tablespoons fish sauce
1	large zucchini
4	scallions, sliced
1	(13.5-ounce) can full-fat coconut milk
2	tablespoons fresh lime juice
1	large avocado, cubed
½	cup cilantro leaves, finely chopped (optional)

CREAMY BEEF AND MUSHROOM SOUP

This soup recipe calls for roasting the mushrooms before adding them to the soup, which gives the soup a richer flavor. If you would rather this be more like a stew than a soup, reduce the broth by about half.

SERVES 6

- 3 tablespoons fat of choice (bacon fat, tallow, or lard recommended)
- 1½ pounds beef stew meat, cubed
- 1 beef soup bone (optional, but recommended)

  Kosher salt and ground black pepper
- 6 cups beef bone broth, homemade (page 35) or store-bought
- 2 tablespoons Primal-cesterershire Sauce (page 264) or apple cider vinegar
- 1 medium onion, chopped
- 2 stalks celery, sliced

MACRONUTRIENTS PER SERVING
(WITH TAPIOCA STARCH)

CALORIES: 658

FAT: 53 G/477 CALORIES

CARBOHYDRATE: 12 G/
48 CALORIES

PROTEIN: 35 G/140 CALORIES

1. In a large soup pot, heat 2 tablespoons of the fat over medium-high heat. Season the meat and soup bone (if using) generously with salt and pepper. When the fat starts to smoke, brown the meat and the bone, 3 to 4 minutes per side. Work in batches to avoid crowding the pan, adding more fat if necessary. (To save time, you can brown half the meat in a separate pan.) Remove the browned meat to a bowl.

2. Pour 1 cup of broth into the pot and deglaze, scraping the bottom of the pot with a wooden spoon to release any browned bits stuck on the bottom. (If you used a second pan, deglaze that with some of the broth, too, and pour the liquid into the soup pot.)

3. Return the meat and bones to the pot, along with any juices that collected in the bowl. Add the rest of the broth, along with the primal-cesterershire sauce, onion, celery, garlic, thyme, and bay leaves. Stir well. Bring the mixture to a boil, reduce to a simmer, and set a timer for 1 hour.

4. When the soup has been simmering for about an hour, preheat the oven to 400°F.

5. Toss the mushrooms with the avocado oil, ½ teaspoon kosher salt, and ¼ teaspoon pepper. Spread them on a large, heavy rimmed baking sheet. Roast them in the oven for 30 minutes, stirring once.

6. When the mushrooms are done, carefully ladle about ¾ cup broth from the soup pot into a blender. Add 2 cups of the roasted mushrooms and the tapioca starch (if using). Blend until smooth.

7. Remove the soup bone, bay leaves, and thyme stems (most of the leaves will have detached) from the pot. Stir the slurry from the blender into the soup. Stir in the rest of the mushrooms and the crème fraîche (if using). Taste and adjust the salt. Simmer until heated through, another 5 to 10 minutes. Serve hot.

4	cloves garlic, chopped
3	sprigs fresh thyme
2	bay leaves
24	ounces cremini mushrooms, quartered
2	tablespoons avocado oil
1	tablespoon tapioca starch (optional)
¾	cup full-fat crème fraîche, heavy whipping cream, or coconut milk (optional)

SAUSAGE AND SHRIMP SOUP

With its Cajun seasoning, this soup is reminiscent of gumbo, the classic Creole dish, but without the roux (made with white flour) that usually thickens gumbo.

SERVES 4

4   slices sugar-free bacon, cut in half

4   links fully cooked sugar-free Italian chicken sausage (hot or sweet), cut into ½-inch-thick slices

6   leaves Swiss chard, ribs and leaves separated

½   cup chopped onion

1   stalk celery, finely sliced

4   cloves garlic, minced

5   cups chicken bone broth, homemade (page 35) or store-bought

1   tablespoon Cajun Seasoning (page 254)

½   teaspoon sea salt

½   teaspoon ground black pepper

2   bay leaves

12   large shrimp, peeled, deveined, and tails removed

MACRONUTRIENTS PER SERVING

CALORIES: 348

FAT: 21 G/191 CALORIES

CARBOHYDRATE: 8 G/ 34 CALORIES

PROTEIN: 30 G/121 CALORIES

1. Heat a soup pot over medium heat and cook the bacon, flipping occasionally, until crispy. Remove to a plate and set aside.

2. Add the sliced sausage to the bacon fat in the pan and brown all over, about 3 minutes per side. Use a slotted spoon to remove the sausage to a bowl and set aside.

3. Slice the chard ribs. Add the chard ribs, onion, and celery to the pot and sauté the veggies until they start to soften, about 3 minutes. Add the garlic and sauté 1 minute more.

4. Deglaze the pot with about ½ cup of the broth, using a wooden spoon to scrape up any browned bits stuck to the bottom. Add the Cajun seasoning, salt, pepper, bay leaves, and the rest of the chicken broth and bring to a boil. Reduce the heat and simmer for 15 minutes to allow the flavors to meld. Discard the bay leaves.

5. Chop the chard leaves into small pieces. Stir them into the soup along with the cooked sausage and any reserved juices. Simmer until the chard is tender, about 10 minutes.

6. Add the shrimp. Return the soup to a simmer and cook until the shrimp are barely opaque all the way through, about 5 minutes (do not overcook or they will be rubbery).

7. Ladle the soup into individual serving bowls. Crumble the cooked bacon and sprinkle it on top of the soup.

CURRIED CHICKEN SALAD

This chicken salad just gets better as it sits in the fridge. Use rotisserie chicken to save time, and adjust the amount of curry powder based on how spicy you want the final dish.

SERVES 4

- ¼ cup avocado oil mayonnaise
- ¼ cup plain full-fat Greek yogurt
- 1 tablespoon curry powder
- ¼ teaspoon ground cinnamon
- 2 teaspoons fresh lime juice
- ¼ teaspoon sea salt
- ⅛ teaspoon ground black pepper
- 1 pound cooked chicken, cubed
- 2 stalks celery with leaves, thinly sliced
- 2 scallions, chopped
- 2 tablespoons chopped fresh cilantro leaves
- ¼ cup slivered almonds
- 2 tablespoons chopped cashews

Lettuce leaves, for serving

1. In a medium bowl, stir together the mayo, yogurt, curry powder, cinnamon, lime juice, salt, and pepper. Add the chicken, celery, scallions, and cilantro. Stir very well to combine. Ideally, refrigerate the mixture for at least 1 hour to chill.

2. Right before serving, stir in the slivered almonds. Sprinkle the cashews over top. Serve with lettuce leaves on the side for wrapping.

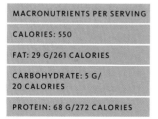

MACRONUTRIENTS PER SERVING

CALORIES: 550

FAT: 29 G/261 CALORIES

CARBOHYDRATE: 5 G/ 20 CALORIES

PROTEIN: 68 G/272 CALORIES

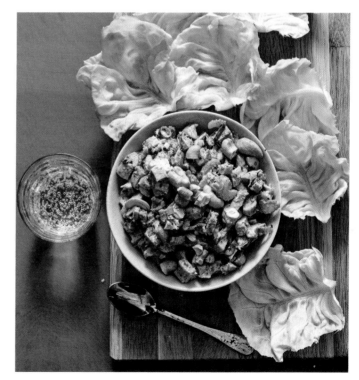

SESAME ASPARAGUS ZOODLE SALAD

This light salad is lovely paired with some simple grilled chicken or fish. It offers a nice alternative to creamy slaws and side dishes.

SERVES 6

2 large zucchini

1 tablespoon + ½ teaspoon kosher salt

1 pound asparagus (choose thick spears), woody ends cut off

3 tablespoons coconut aminos or tamari

1½ tablespoons sesame oil

1½ tablespoons extra-virgin olive oil

1 tablespoon finely grated fresh ginger

2 tablespoons toasted sesame seeds

MACRONUTRIENTS PER SERVING

CALORIES: 114

FAT: 8 G/72 CALORIES

CARBOHYDRATE: 8 G/ 32 CALORIES

PROTEIN: 4 G/16 CALORIES

1. Cut the zucchini into noodles using a spiralizer or other noodle-cutting tool. Place the zucchini noodles in a sieve in your sink or over a large bowl. Toss the noodles with ½ teaspoon kosher salt and leave them to drain.

2. In a pot, combine 4 cups water and 1 tablespoon kosher salt and bring it to a boil over high heat.

3. Meanwhile, make the asparagus noodles: Lay one asparagus spear at a time on a cutting board. Holding it by the tip, place a vegetable peeler just below the tip and draw it down the length of the spear to create a thin ribbon. Turn the asparagus over and do the same down the other side, avoiding the tip. Continue until only a thin strip is left. (When the spear becomes thin, place it on the handle of a wooden spoon or spatula to prop it up. This will allow you to use the peeler without it hitting the cutting board.) Use a knife to cut off the last ribbon from the tip. Collect the ribbons in one bowl and the tips in another.

4. When the water comes to a boil, drop in the asparagus tips only and boil for 2 minutes. Drain and run the tips under cold water to stop the cooking.

5. Use a wooden spoon or a spatula to gently press down on the zucchini noodles to squeeze the liquid out of them. Stir and press again. Repeat several more times until no liquid runs out. Place the zucchini noodles in a clean kitchen towel.

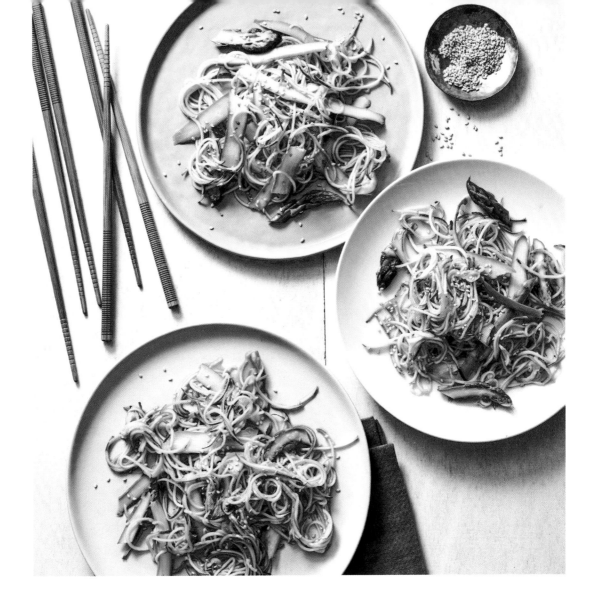

Roll up the towel and press down gently to squeeze even more moisture out of them. Transfer the zucchini noodles to a serving bowl. Add the shaved asparagus ribbons.

6. In a small bowl, whisk together the coconut aminos, sesame oil, olive oil, and ginger. Pour about two-thirds of the dressing over the zucchini and asparagus noodles and toss well. Arrange the asparagus tips on top of the salad and drizzle with the remaining dressing. Sprinkle with the sesame seeds and serve immediately.

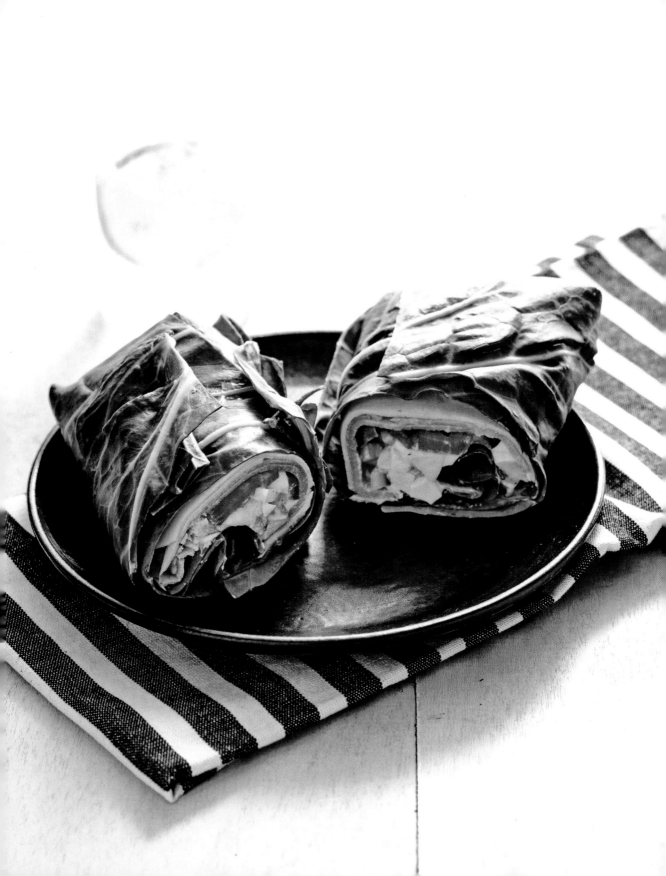

HANDHELD CHEF SALAD

Collard green wraps are a convenient option for keto-friendly lunches. Lettuce or Swiss chard also work, but collards hold up the best. This variation on a collard green wrap takes the classic American chef salad and makes it portable.

SERVES 2

4 large collard green leaves

2 hard-boiled eggs

1½ tablespoons avocado oil mayonnaise

1½ tablespoons keto-friendly ranch dressing or Wild Ranch Dressing (page 266)

½ cucumber, seeded and finely diced

4 thin slices deli turkey

4 thin slices deli ham

1 Roma (plum) tomato, sliced as thinly as possible

Ground black pepper

MACRONUTRIENTS PER SERVING*
CALORIES: 303
FAT: 21 G/189 CALORIES
CARBOHYDRATE: 10 G/ 40 CALORIES
PROTEIN: 21 G/84 CALORIES

* Macros based on using Primal Kitchen Ranch Dressing.

1. Use a sharp knife to remove the thick stems from the collard greens, but keep each leaf intact as much as possible.

2. In a small bowl, use a fork to mash the eggs. Add the mayo and ranch dressing. Use the fork to stir them together. It is okay if the egg mixture remains somewhat chunky like egg salad. Stir in the cucumber.

3. To assemble each wrap, lay out 2 collard greens stem end to stem end, overlapping about 3 inches. Place 2 slices of turkey and 2 slices of ham in the middle (there should be an inch or more of collard green still showing at each end). Place slices of tomato in a line down the middle. Spoon half the egg salad over the tomatoes. Top with a pinch of pepper.

4. Roll up the collard greens like a burrito, folding the collard greens in as you roll. Secure with one or two toothpicks. Repeat for the second wrap. Optionally cut each wrap in half with a sharp knife to serve.

LOADED FAUX-TATO SOUP

Sometimes it feels like a keto diet is really a cauliflower diet—cauliflower shows up everywhere! Even if you're a little over cauliflower rice and cauliflower pizza crust, give this recipe a try. The addition of a parsnip—an ingredient some keto dieters might unnecessarily avoid—plus the step of roasting the vegetables takes this way beyond a boring cauliflower soup. You would swear this really is loaded baked potato soup (except it's better)!

SERVES 6

2   medium heads cauliflower, cut into small florets

1   small parsnip, peeled and cut into ½-inch cubes

3   tablespoons avocado oil

    Kosher salt

6   slices sugar-free bacon (optional), or 1 tablespoon bacon fat or avocado oil

2   cups chicken bone broth, homemade (page 35) or store-bought

1   cup heavy whipping cream

    Ground black pepper

6   tablespoons full-fat sour cream

¾   cup shredded sharp cheddar cheese

    Finely chopped fresh chives, for garnish

1. Preheat the oven to 425°F.

2. Toss the cauliflower and parsnip with the avocado oil and ¾ teaspoon kosher salt. Divide the veggies between two heavy rimmed baking sheets. Roast them in the oven until lightly browned and crisp-tender, 15 minutes.

3. Meanwhile (if using bacon), in the soup pot you will use for the soup, cook the bacon in two batches until crispy. Set the cooked bacon aside. Pour off all but about 1 tablespoon of the bacon fat from the pot. (Save the remaining bacon fat to use in a different recipe.) Use about ½ cup of the broth to deglaze the pot, using a wooden spoon to scrape up the browned bits that are stuck to the bottom. Remove from the heat.

4. When the cauliflower and parsnips are roasted, transfer them to the soup pot and set over medium-high. Add the bacon fat or avocado oil (if not using bacon). Pour in the rest of the chicken broth, bring to a boil, cover, reduce the heat, and simmer until the vegetables are very soft, 10 minutes.

5. Uncover and stir in the heavy cream and ½ teaspoon pepper. Heat just until hot.

6. Remove from the heat. Use an immersion blender to blend the soup until smooth. (Alternatively, working in batches, *carefully* transfer the soup to a regular blender and blend it until smooth. Do not overfill the blender.) Taste the soup and adjust the salt and pepper. Stir in half the cheddar.

7. Ladle the soup into bowls. Top each serving with 1 table-spoon sour cream, 1 tablespoon cheddar, and a sprinkling of fresh chives. Crumble 1 piece of the bacon on top of each bowl of soup if desired. Serve hot.

Note: If you can't find parsnip, use daikon radish instead, or simply add another 1½ to 2 cups of cauliflower florets. If you are allowing a bit more carbohydrates, you can also substitute a white potato or a Japanese sweet potato for some healthy nutrient-dense carbs.

CRAB SALAD RÉMOULADE

Rémoulade is a creamy dressing or sauce that is French in origin, but it has become emblematic of the Cajun cooking you'll find, especially in Louisiana, in the US. Here it forms the base of a crab salad. You can use either fresh or frozen lump crabmeat, just make sure it is crab and not krab!

SERVES 4

½ cup avocado oil mayonnaise

2 tablespoons Dijon mustard (whole-grain recommended)

½ teaspoon prepared horseradish

½ teaspoon Cajun Seasoning (page 253)

½ teaspoon sweet paprika

¼ teaspoon garlic powder

⅛ teaspoon cayenne pepper (optional)

1 teaspoon fresh lemon juice

1 pound lump crabmeat (not imitation)

1 stalk celery with leaves, finely chopped

2 scallions, finely chopped

8 cups arugula

2 avocados, sliced

1 lemon, cut into wedges

1. In a bowl, combine the mayo, mustard, horseradish, Cajun seasoning, paprika, garlic powder, cayenne (if using), and lemon juice. Add the crabmeat, celery, and scallions. Stir very well to combine. (*Optional*: Refrigerate the salad to chill.)

2. To serve, place 2 cups arugula on each salad plate. Arrange ½ sliced avocado on top. Scoop one-quarter of the salad mixture on top of the avocado. Serve with a lemon wedge.

MACRONUTRIENTS PER SERVING
CALORIES: 293
FAT: 26 G/236 CALORIES
CARBOHYDRATE: 10 G/ 40 CALORIES
PROTEIN: 9 G/36 CALORIES

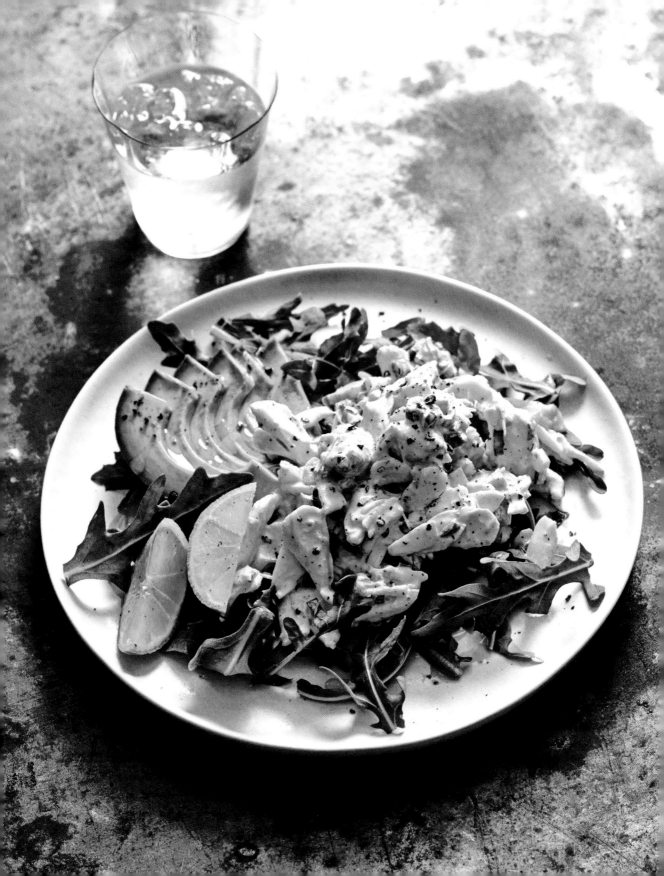

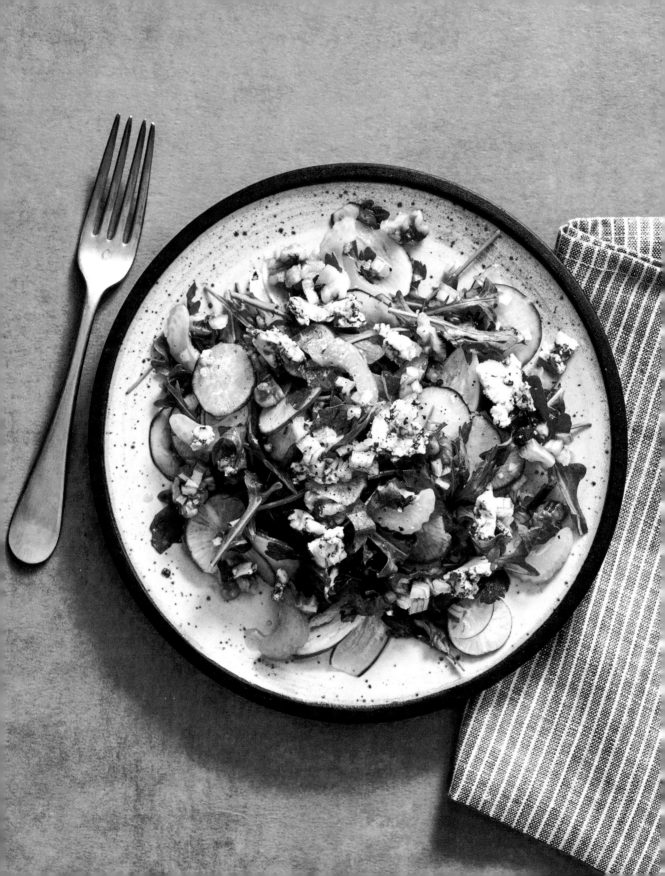

RADISH CRUNCH SALAD WITH CITRUS VINAIGRETTE

Radishes are so underappreciated! They are excellent both raw and cooked (see the Butter-Braised Radishes on page 201). Check your local grocery store or farmers' market to find different sizes and varieties. See if you can find watermelon radishes or other varieties that have colors and patterns on the inside to add visual interest to this salad.

SERVES 4

FOR THE DRESSING

- ¼ cup extra-virgin olive oil
- Grated zest and juice of 1 Meyer lemon or 1 small regular lemon
- Juice of 1 small lime
- 1 small shallot, finely minced
- ¼ teaspoon sea salt
- ⅛ teaspoon ground black pepper

FOR THE SALAD

- 8 cups arugula, or other salad greens such as baby kale or spinach
- ½ cup packed fresh parsley leaves, chopped
- 1 small bunch radishes, thinly sliced
- 2 stalks celery with leaves, thinly sliced
- ½ cup chopped pecans or walnuts
- ½ cup crumbled blue cheese, feta, or goat cheese

1. For the dressing: In a jar with a tight-fitting lid, shake together the oil, lemon zest, lemon juice, lime juice, shallot, salt, and pepper until well combined.

2. For the salad: In a bowl, toss the arugula and parsley with half the dressing. Divide the greens among four salad bowls. Arrange the sliced radishes on top, then sprinkle with celery, pecans, and blue cheese. Drizzle the remaining dressing evenly over the salads. Serve immediately.

MACRONUTRIENTS PER SERVING
CALORIES: 305
FAT: 29 G/257 CALORIES
CARBOHYDRATE: 9 G/ 34 CALORIES
PROTEIN: 7 G/28 CALORIES

ENTRÉES

BONE-IN BUTTER CHICKEN

This recipe is a must-try! Most butter chicken recipes call for boneless, skinless chicken, but whenever possible, heed the words of Dr. Cate Shanahan, who calls meat on the bone one of the pillars of "deep nutrition." You can also use chicken breasts, but thighs are recommended. Serve with Triple-Coconut Cauliflower Rice (page 165).

SERVES 6

6   large bone-in chicken thighs, skin removed

Sea salt and ground black pepper

1   tablespoon avocado oil

4   tablespoons ghee or unsalted butter

1   small onion, diced

3   cloves garlic, finely chopped

2   teaspoons chili powder

2   teaspoons garam masala

2   teaspoons ground ginger

2   teaspoons ground turmeric

1   cup chicken bone broth, homemade (page 35) or store-bought

2   tablespoons tomato paste

2   cups heavy whipping cream or full-fat coconut milk

MACRONUTRIENTS PER SERVING
CALORIES: 517
FAT: 44 G/393 CALORIES
CARBOHYDRATE: 8 G/ 32 CALORIES
PROTEIN: 24 G/96 CALORIES

1. Generously season the chicken thighs with salt and pepper. Heat a large skillet over medium-high heat. Add the avocado oil and 2 tablespoons of the ghee and when hot, place the chicken thighs meat side down and cook undisturbed for 5 minutes. Do this in two batches if necessary to avoid crowding the pan. Flip and cook another 2 minutes. Remove the chicken thighs to a bowl to catch any liquid.

2. Reduce the heat to medium. Add the remaining 2 tablespoons ghee to the skillet. When hot, add the onion and sauté for 3 minutes, until soft. Add the garlic and sauté 1 minute more. Add the chili powder, garam masala, ginger, and turmeric and cook, stirring constantly, for 30 seconds. Do not let the spices burn.

3. Pour in ½ cup of the chicken broth and use a wooden spoon or silicone spatula to scrape up the browned bits stuck to the bottom. Add the remaining broth and continue scraping. When the pan is fully deglazed, return the chicken thighs and any accumulated juices to the pan. Bring to a boil, reduce to a simmer, and cook uncovered for 15 minutes, flipping the chicken occasionally to coat with the sauce.

4. Spoon a few tablespoons of the hot cooking liquid into a small bowl. Whisk the tomato paste into it, then pour it back into the skillet. Stir in the cream and simmer until the chicken is completely cooked through and the sauce is thickened,

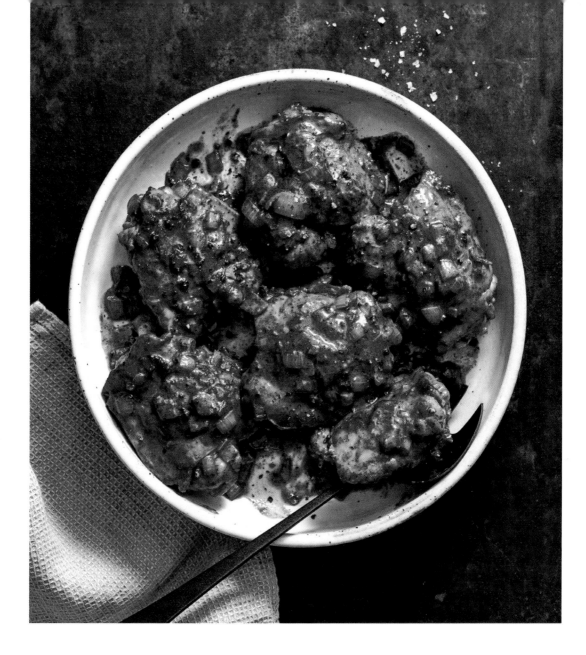

TIP: If you remove the skin from the thighs yourself, save it, along with the leftover bones, in your freezer to make bone broth with later.

another 15 minutes, continuing to flip the chicken every few minutes.

5. Taste the sauce and adjust the salt and pepper. Serve the chicken with the sauce poured over top.

TACO TURKEY BURGERS

For this recipe, look for whole green chiles in the pickled and preserved foods section of the grocery store. Chopped green chiles or even a mild green salsa will work, too.

SERVES 4

1½ pounds ground turkey (thigh or breast)

1 tablespoon Taco Seasoning Blend (page 253)

¼ cup canned chopped green chiles

2 tablespoons avocado oil

Sea salt and ground black pepper

4 canned fire-roasted whole green chiles (or an additional ½ cup chopped green chiles)

4 slices pepper jack cheese

TOPPINGS/ADDITIONS (OPTIONAL)

Sliced avocado or guacamole

Full-fat sour cream

Prepared salsa

Collard greens or Swiss chard for wrapping

1. In a large bowl, combine the ground turkey, taco seasoning, and ¼ cup chopped green chiles. Form the turkey mixture into 4 patties about ½ inch thick.

2. In a large skillet, heat the avocado oil over medium-high heat. Generously season the patties on both sides with salt and pepper. Place the patties in the pan and cover with the lid. Cook on the first side for 5 minutes. Flip and cook uncovered until the burgers are cooked through, 5 minutes more.

3. Meanwhile, position an oven rack 4 to 6 inches below the broiler. Preheat the broiler to low.

4. Use a spatula to transfer the patties to a broilerproof pan. Cut the whole green chiles in half crosswise and place them on top of the patties (or sprinkle the chopped green chiles evenly over the patties). Place a slice of cheese on top of each patty, covering the chiles.

5. Broil the patties, watching carefully, until the cheese starts to bubble and brown, about 2 minutes.

6. Remove the burgers from the oven and top with any of the optional toppings if desired. Optionally wrap the burgers in collard greens or Swiss chard leaves to serve.

MACRONUTRIENTS PER SERVING (NO TOPPINGS)

CALORIES: 522

FAT: 33 G/298 CALORIES

CARBOHYDRATE: 5 G/ 20 CALORIES

PROTEIN: 52 G/209 CALORIES

INSTANT POT RIBS

Slow-smoking ribs is obviously great, but let's be real, some-times we're hungry *now*. Instant Pot to the rescue!

SERVES 4

1   large or 2 small racks baby back ribs (2½ to 3 pounds)

2   teaspoons kosher salt

2   teaspoons ground black pepper

1½   tablespoons Choco-Chili Rub (page 253)

1   cup water

Keto "BBQ Sauce" (optional; page 258)

MACRONUTRIENTS PER SERVING (NO SAUCE)
CALORIES: 550
FAT: 37 G/333 CALORIES
CARBOHYDRATE: 2 G/ 8 CALORIES
PROTEIN: 52 G/208 CALORIES

1. Remove the silverskin from the bone side of the ribs by grabbing the edge with a paper towel and pulling it away from the ribs.

2. Generously salt and pepper both sides of the ribs. Sprinkle the rub all over the ribs and press it into the meat. (This step can be done the day before if you want your ribs to be extra flavorful.)

3. Place the water into the Instant Pot. Place the metal steam rack/trivet in the pot. Arrange the ribs on the rack. You might need to cut the ribs in half to fit.

4. Secure the lid and set the steam release valve to Sealing. Press the "Meat" button and set the cook time to 25 minutes.

5. When the Instant Pot beeps, allow the pressure to release naturally for 10 minutes, then carefully switch the steam release valve to Venting. When fully released, open and trans-fer the ribs to a heavy rimmed baking sheet or broiling pan.

6. Position the oven rack 6 inches from the broiler. Heat the broiler to low.

7. Broil the ribs until the surface crisps, about 2 minutes. *Optional:* Brush the BBQ sauce all over the top of the ribs and return to the broiler for another minute. Serve with any remaining sauce on the side.

CHOCO CHICKEN

This recipe was originally inspired by molé chicken, which, although delicious, is not keto-friendly. Serve this over Basic Cauliflower Rice (page 37).

SERVES 4

3 tablespoons unsweetened cocoa powder

2 teaspoons ground cinnamon

1 teaspoon dried oregano

1 teaspoon ancho chile powder (see Notes)

½ teaspoon ground cumin

½ teaspoon ground coriander

½ teaspoon sea salt

MACRONUTRIENTS PER SERVING

CALORIES: 478

FAT: 38 G/338 CALORIES

CARBOHYDRATE: 11 G/ 44 CALORIES

PROTEIN: 31 G/124 CALORIES

1. For the spice mixture: In a small bowl, combine the cocoa powder, cinnamon, oregano, ancho chile powder, cumin, coriander, and the salt.

2. For the chicken: Season the chicken thighs with the salt and pepper. In a heavy skillet, melt the coconut oil over medium-high heat. When the oil is hot, place the chicken in the pan and cook it 3 to 4 minutes per side to lightly brown the chicken. Remove it to a plate (it will not be totally cooked through yet, which is fine).

3. Reduce the heat to medium under the skillet. Add the onion and sauté, stirring frequently, until the onions are very soft and starting to brown, about 6 minutes. Add the garlic and sauté 1 minute more.

4. Add the spice mixture and stir quickly to coat the onions. Add ½ cup of the broth and deglaze the pan by using a wooden spoon to scrape any browned bits stuck to the bottom. Add the remaining ½ cup broth and the coconut milk. Bring the sauce to a boil, stirring constantly.

5. Return the chicken thighs and any accumulated juices to the pan, flipping to coat both sides with sauce. Reduce the heat to a simmer and cook, flipping the chicken occasionally, to let the flavors develop and the sauce thicken, about 25 minutes.

6. Remove the chicken from the pan and when cool enough to handle, shred the chicken. *Optional*: Use an immersion blender to blend the sauce in the pan until smooth.

7. Stir the shredded chicken into the sauce. Simmer 5 minutes more. Divide the chicken among four plates or bowls and serve it with additional sauce from the skillet spooned over the top.

Notes

- Do not omit the ancho chile powder in this recipe. If you do not have any on hand, you can substitute chili powder or chipotle powder (be aware that chipotle is considerably spicier), but it's worth a run to the grocery store to get ancho if you can.
- Thighs are recommended, but you can substitute chicken breast in this recipe. We recommend if the breasts are thick that you pound them thinner before cooking, otherwise you might need to increase the simmering time in step 5.

FOR THE CHICKEN

1½	pounds boneless, skinless chicken thighs (see Notes)
¾	teaspoon sea salt
½	teaspoon ground black pepper
2	tablespoons coconut oil
½	large onion, chopped
2	cloves garlic, chopped
1	cup chicken bone broth, homemade (page 35) or store-bought
1	(13.5-ounce) can full-fat coconut milk

CRISPY PORK BELLY BITES

These pork belly bites are awesome for a bunch of reasons. First, they involve no advanced planning—no marinating and no overnight air-drying like in many pork belly recipes. Second, they cook in a third of the time of typical pork belly roasts. Because of how they are prepared, they also tend to be a little bit firmer than when you roast a whole pork belly. If you haven't been keen on pork belly in the past because of its somewhat gelatinous mouthfeel, give this version a try!

SERVES 4

1   pork belly (about 2 pounds)

1   teaspoon sea salt

1   teaspoon Chinese five-spice powder

FOR THE DIPPING SAUCE

¼   cup tamari or coconut aminos

1   tablespoon + 1 teaspoon sesame oil

½   teaspoon ground ginger

1. Preheat the oven to 450°F.

2. Heat your biggest cast-iron or other ovenproof skillet (see Note) over medium-high heat until very hot, 4 minutes or so.

3. While the skillet heats, pat the skin side of the pork belly dry and rub the salt all over the skin. When the skillet is hot, place the pork belly skin side down in the dry skillet and cook undisturbed for 4 minutes. If the pork belly is too long to fit in the skillet, cut it in half and do this step in two batches.

4. Remove from the heat and carefully transfer the pork belly to a cutting board, skin side down. When cool enough to handle, rub the Chinese five-spice powder into the meat side. Use a very sharp knife to cut the pork belly into strips about ½ inch wide.

5. Arrange the pork belly slices in a single layer in the hot skillet. Do not pour off any fat in the skillet. It is okay if the strips overlap somewhat because they will shrink when cooking. (But if they will not all fit, see Note, making sure to save the fat in the skillet.)

6. Place the skillet in the hot oven and cook for 15 minutes.

7. While the pork belly cooks, make the dipping sauce. In a small jar with a tight-fitting lid, combine the tamari, sesame oil, and ground ginger and shake vigorously to combine.

CREAMY SAUTÉED LIVER

Sometimes recipes are designed to highlight the taste of liver (like the Chopped Liver recipe on page 210), while others aim to hide it (like the Offal Bacon Burgers on page 145). This recipe is somewhere in the middle. Liver is the star, but the creamy sauce might be enough to sway someone who is on the fence about liver. Of course, if you're a liver lover already, this is for you.

SERVES 4

1¼	teaspoons ground coriander
¾	teaspoon ground turmeric
¼	teaspoon ground cumin
¾	teaspoon kosher salt
½	teaspoon ground black pepper
2	tablespoons coconut oil
½	cup diced onion
3	cloves garlic, minced
1	pound liver (beef or pork), cut into thin strips
¼	cup filtered water or broth
1	tablespoon coconut aminos or tamari
1½	tablespoons almond butter
1	cup full-fat coconut milk

MACRONUTRIENTS PER SERVING

CALORIES: 429

FAT: 26 G/237 CALORIES

CARBOHYDRATE: 13 G/ 51 CALORIES

PROTEIN: 35 G/142 CALORIES

1. In a small bowl, mix together the coriander, turmeric, cumin, salt, and pepper. Set both aside.

2. In a large skillet, heat 1 tablespoon of the coconut oil over medium heat. Add the onion and garlic and cook until just softening, 3 to 4 minutes. Add the spices to the onion and cook another minute, stirring constantly. Remove the onions to a bowl.

3. Increase the heat to medium-high and add the remaining 1 tablespoon coconut oil to the pan. When it is hot, add the liver. Cook the liver for about 2 minutes, then stir the onions back in. Add the water and deglaze the skillet, scraping the bottom very well with a wooden spoon to scrape up the browned bits. Cook for another 3 minutes.

4. In a small bowl, mix together the coconut aminos and almond butter. Whisk in the coconut milk. Pour the mixture into the skillet and stir very well, scraping the bottom of the pan again. Allow the mixture to come to a boil, then reduce the heat to a low simmer. Cover the pan and simmer for 15 minutes to allow the flavors to meld. Serve hot.

MEATZA PIZZA STUFFED PEPPERS

Lots of keto pizza recipes call for some sort of crust substitute, but it's never the same as the original. Who needs pizza crust anyway? The toppings are where it's at, and this recipe is full of them.

SERVES 4

2	teaspoons pork lard or fat of your choice
½	small onion, diced
2	cloves garlic, minced
½	pound ground beef
½	pound fresh Italian sausage links (sweet or hot), casings removed
½	teaspoon dried oregano
½	teaspoon sea salt
¼	teaspoon ground black pepper
1	tablespoon tomato paste
2	large bell peppers, any color
8	ounces fresh mozzarella cheese, shredded or thinly sliced
¼	cup shredded Parmesan cheese
8	thin pepperoni slices

MACRONUTRIENTS PER SERVING

CALORIES: 566

FAT: 39 G/353 CALORIES

CARBOHYDRATE: 12 G/ 46 CALORIES

PROTEIN: 39 G/158 CALORIES

1. Preheat the oven to 425°F.

2. In a skillet, heat the lard over medium heat. Add the onion and sauté until just soft, about 3 minutes. Add the garlic and sauté for 1 minute more.

3. Crumble in the beef and sausage. Stir in the oregano, salt, and black pepper. Cook, using a fork or meat chopper to break up the meat, until almost no pink remains, about 6 minutes. Stir in the tomato paste and continue to cook until no pink remains. Taste and adjust the salt and pepper.

4. Halve the bell peppers lengthwise, through the stem. Cut out the ribs and seeds without puncturing the pepper. Place the peppers in a single layer in a baking dish that fits them snugly enough that they do not roll around. If you want the peppers to be very soft in the final product, place them in the hot oven for 5 minutes. Otherwise, proceed to the next step.

5. Divide the mozzarella into 8 equal portions. Fill each half pepper halfway with the meat mixture. Top with half the mozzarella. Fill the rest of the way with meat. Top with the remaining mozzarella, the Parmesan, and 2 pepperoni slices per pepper. (If you have meat mixture left over, save it for tomorrow's breakfast omelet!)

6. Bake the peppers until they are soft and the cheese is bubbly, about 20 minutes. (*Optional*: Heat the broiler to low and broil for 1 to 2 minutes to brown the top further.) Remove from the oven and serve hot.

Mix it up! Customize these to match your favorite pizza. Add bacon or mushrooms to the ground meat (decrease the amount of meat accordingly), or top with black olives or anchovies! You can also add more tomato paste to the filling, but you'll want to calculate the macros to watch the carbs.

ONE-PAN CHICKEN AND VEGGIES

Who doesn't love a one-pan meal! You can throw this recipe together in a matter of minutes, especially if you chop the vegetables ahead of time or buy prechopped vegetables from the grocery store. It's a perfect weeknight dinner for a busy family.

SERVES 6

2	pounds boneless or 2½ pounds bone-in chicken breasts
1	tablespoon salted butter, ghee, or fat of choice, melted
2	teaspoons Italian Seasoning Blend (page 254)
1	teaspoon kosher salt
1	small onion, cut into 1-inch chunks
1	red or yellow bell pepper, cut into 1-inch chunks
1	small eggplant, cut into ¾-inch cubes
1	cup grape tomatoes
2½	tablespoons avocado oil
1½	cups shredded mozzarella cheese (optional)

1. Preheat the oven to 425°F.

2. Place the chicken breasts on a heavy rimmed baking sheet. Pour the melted butter over them, then season them with 1 teaspoon of the Italian seasoning and ½ teaspoon salt. If you're using bone-in chicken breasts, place in the oven for 10 minutes before adding the vegetables in step 4.

3. In a large bowl, combine the onion, bell pepper, eggplant, and tomatoes. Add the avocado oil and the remaining 1 teaspoon Italian seasoning and ½ teaspoon salt and stir to coat.

4. Arrange the vegetables on the baking sheet around the chicken breasts. Roast until the internal temperature of the chicken reaches 165°F, 25 to 30 minutes.

5. Remove the pan from the oven and let the chicken rest for a few minutes. At this point you can slice the chicken breasts and plate them alongside the vegetables, or . . .

6. *Optional:* Position an oven rack 4 to 6 inches from the broiler. Heat the broiler to high.

MACRONUTRIENTS PER SERVING
(WITH CHEESE)

CALORIES: 402

FAT: 21 G/189 CALORIES

CARBOHYDRATE: 8 G/
32 CALORIES

PROTEIN: 43 G/172 CALORIES

7. Remove the chicken to a cutting board and cut the meat into roughly bite-size pieces. Return the meat to the baking pan and use a spoon or spatula to gently toss it with the vegetables. Crowd the chicken and vegetables in the center of the baking sheet in a single layer. Sprinkle the mozzarella evenly over the top. Broil until the cheese melts and starts to brown, 1 to 2 minutes. Keep an eye on it!

8. To serve, use the sharp edge of a metal spatula to divide the chicken and vegetables into 6 equal servings. Slide the spatula under each serving and transfer it to a plate. Serve hot.

Mix it up!

- Instead of Italian seasoning, use Greek Seasoning Blend (page 253) and substitute ½ cup feta cheese for ½ cup of the mozzarella.
- Or use Taco Seasoning Blend (page 255) instead, swap the eggplant for mushrooms (cut in half), and use a Mexican shredded cheese blend on top.

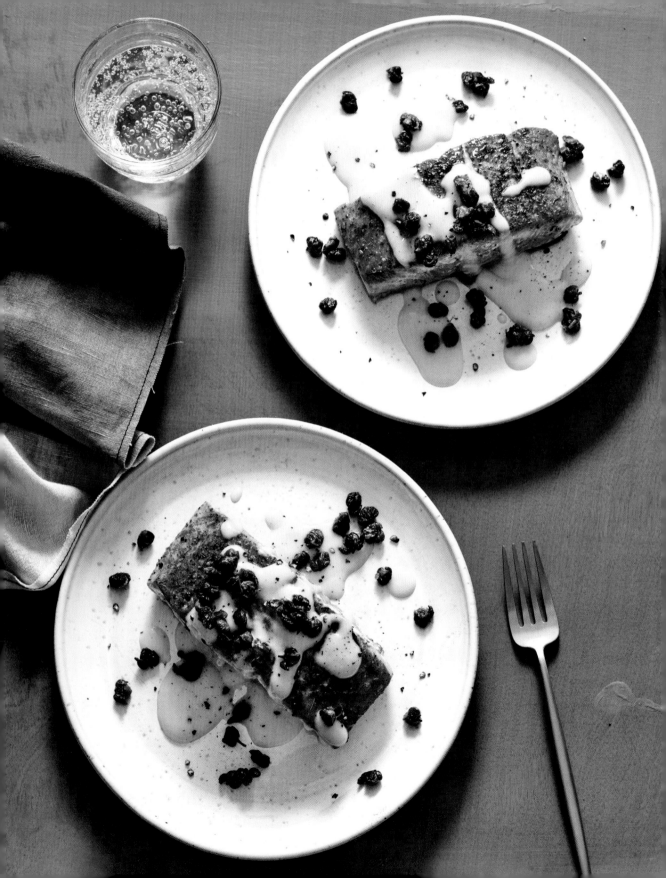

PAN-SEARED SALMON WITH QUICK HOLLANDAISE AND CRISPY CAPERS

This is a great weeknight option because of how quickly it comes together. You can make the hollandaise while the salmon cooks, or you can even make it the night before.

SERVES 4

4   skin-on salmon fillets (4 ounces each)

¾   teaspoon Cajun Seasoning (page 253)

¼   teaspoon sea salt

2   tablespoons avocado oil

2   tablespoons capers, drained

      Quick Hollandaise (page 257), made with the optional Cajun Seasoning

MACRONUTRIENTS PER SERVING

CALORIES: 511

FAT: 42 G/382 CALORIES

CARBOHYDRATE: 1 G/ 3 CALORIES

PROTEIN: 31 G/125 CALORIES

1. Pat the salmon fillets with a clean kitchen towel and check for bones. Season the flesh side with the Cajun seasoning and salt.

2. Pour the avocado oil into the bottom of a skillet large enough to hold the salmon. Swirl the skillet to coat the bottom. Add the salmon to the COLD skillet skin side up. Set the skillet over medium-high heat and sear the salmon for 3 minutes without disturbing. (This is a good time to start the hollandaise sauce if you haven't already.) Gently lift one corner of the salmon to check it; sear for 1 more minute if it doesn't release easily from the pan.

3. Use a spatula to flip the salmon and reduce the heat to medium. Cook uncovered until just barely cooked through, another 4 to 5 minutes. Remove to a plate.

4. Add the drained capers to the pan, taking care in case they spatter. Stir-fry them for about 90 seconds. Remove from the heat.

5. Plate the salmon and top each fillet with a generous dollop of the hollandaise. Sprinkle the crispy capers on top. Serve immediately.

CRÈME FRAÎCHE SPATCHCOCKED CHICKEN WITH CREAMY BRUSSELS SPROUTS

This recipe was inspired by a recipe on Mimi Thorisson's beautiful blog *Manger*, in which she chronicles life and food in the French countryside. Mimi roasts a whole chicken coated with herbed crème fraîche. In the version below, spatchcocked chicken is smothered with crème fraîche and herbes de Provence, a nod to Mimi's French influence. Use Brussels sprouts that are on the smaller side so they become very tender during cooking.

SERVES 6

1   whole chicken (about 4 pounds)

1¼ teaspoons kosher salt
    Ground black pepper

4   cloves garlic—2 pressed or finely minced, 2 roughly chopped

3   tablespoons herbes de Provence (see Note)

1   (7.5-ounce) container crème fraiche (about ¾ cup)

2   cups (8 ounces) Brussels sprouts, trimmed and halved

2   stalks celery with leaves, sliced

1   tablespoon avocado oil

1. Thirty minutes before you intend to start cooking the chicken, remove it from the refrigerator. Place the chicken breast side down on a cutting board. Use sharp kitchen shears to cut down either side of the backbone and remove. Turn the chicken over and press down firmly on the chicken. You will hear a cracking sound and the chicken should lie flat. Season the top and underside with about 1 teaspoon each salt and pepper.

2. In a small bowl, stir together the finely minced garlic, the herbes de Provence, and crème fraiche. Set aside.

3. Place the Brussels sprouts cut side down in a large roasting pan (large enough to hold the spatchcocked chicken). Toss in the sliced celery and chopped garlic. Drizzle the vegetables with the avocado oil and season with the remaining ¼ teaspoon salt and a little more pepper.

4. Preheat the oven to 400°F.

5. Spread about ¼ cup of the crème fraîche mixture over the underside of the chicken. Flip it over and place it skin side up

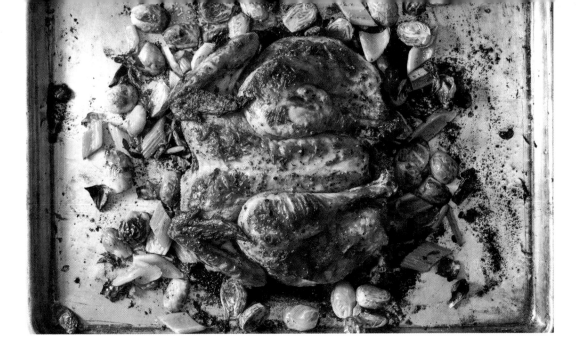

TIP: After spatchcocking the chicken, toss the backbone into your slow cooker, along with the trimmings from your veggies, another clove of garlic, and any other vegetable scraps you have around. Add about 6 cups filtered water, cover, and set the slow cooker to low. After your meal is done, place the leftover bones and skin into the slow cooker. Add more filtered water if needed to cover. Leave the broth to cook on low for 24 to 48 hours, then follow the directions on page 35 to finish.

on top of the vegetables in the roasting pan. Arrange the legs and wings so the bird is lying flat and not hanging over the edge of the roasting pan. Generously coat the chicken with the rest of the crème fraîche mixture, making sure to get into the creases of the wings and thighs.

6. Place the pan in the oven and roast until the internal temperature of a chicken thigh reaches 165°F, 1 hour to 1 hour 15 minutes. Remove the pan from the oven and cover the chicken loosely with foil. Allow it to rest for 10 minutes. Remove the chicken to a cutting board and carve it. Arrange the meat on a warm serving platter. Serve the vegetables in a bowl alongside the chicken.

Note: Herbes de Provence is a seasoning blend that includes, among other things, lavender. This imparts a lovely flavor and aroma to the chicken. However, if you don't have herbes de Provence, you can substitute other fresh or dried herbs of your choosing.

MACRONUTRIENTS PER SERVING
CALORIES: 643
FAT: 40 G/360 CALORIES
CARBOHYDRATE: 3 G/ 12 CALORIES
PROTEIN: 63 G/252 CALORIES

LAMB KOFTA KEBABS WITH TURMERIC DIPPING SAUCE

Kofta is a general term for spiced meatballs that are common in Mediterranean, Middle Eastern, and Southeast Asian cooking. This recipe calls for them to be made into kebabs, but it is equally good if you choose to make the ground meat into meatballs or small patties and pan-cook them. This is delicious served with Shredded Tabbouleh Salad (page 82).

SERVES 4

1 teaspoon kosher salt

4 cloves garlic, pressed or minced

1 pound ground lamb (or use half ground lamb and half ground beef)

2 tablespoons Greek Seasoning Blend (page 253)

¼ cup grated or minced onion

¼ cup fresh parsley leaves, finely chopped

8 metal or bamboo skewers, soaked

1. *Optional but recommended:* Place the salt and garlic in a mortar and pestle and grind the garlic into a paste.

2. In a large bowl, combine the lamb, salt, and garlic (or the garlic paste from the previous step), Greek seasoning, onion, and parsley and mix until thoroughly combined.

3. Divide the meat mixture into 8 equal portions. One at a time, use your hands to roll each portion into a ball. Take a skewer and press it into the middle of each ball. Shape the meat around the skewer, forming it into a flat oval. Place the kofta kebabs on a plate or small baking sheet, cover with a piece of parchment paper, and refrigerate for at least 30 minutes, but up to 24 hours.

4. Meanwhile, make the dipping sauce: In a small food processor or blender, blend together the almond butter, tahini, olive oil, lemon juice, vinegar, garlic, turmeric, salt, and pepper. Add warm water 1 tablespoon at a time until it reaches the desired consistency. Transfer the sauce to a jar and refrigerate until ready to serve.

MACRONUTRIENTS PER SERVING

CALORIES: 538

FAT: 42 G/378 CALORIES

CARBOHYDRATE: 6 G/24 CALORIES

PROTEIN: 35 G/140 CALORIES

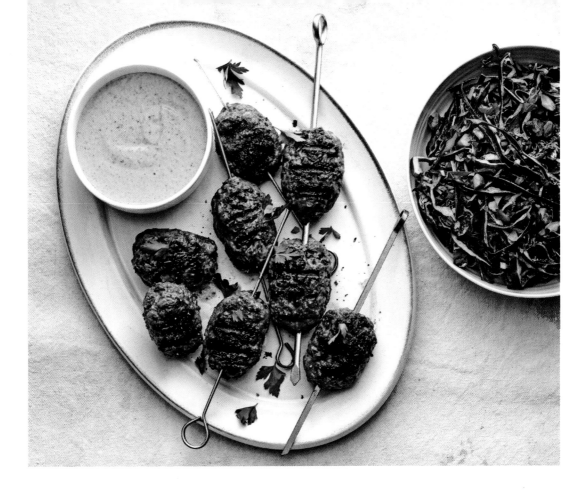

5. Allow the kofta kebabs and dipping sauce to sit at room temperature for 15 minutes.

6. Heat an outdoor grill or indoor grill pan over medium to medium-high heat. Cook the kebabs for 3 minutes per side for medium (depending on thickness). Place on a serving platter. Stir the dipping sauce and transfer it to a serving bowl. Serve the sauce alongside the kebabs.

FOR THE DIPPING SAUCE

- 2 tablespoons almond butter
- 1 tablespoon tahini
- 2 tablespoons extra-virgin olive oil

  Juice of ½ lemon
- 1½ tablespoons apple cider vinegar
- 2 cloves garlic, pressed or finely minced
- ½ teaspoon ground turmeric
- ¼ teaspoon sea salt
- ⅛ teaspoon ground black pepper

  Warm filtered water

BEEF STROGANOFF WITH EGGPLANT "NOODLES"

Usually beef stroganoff is served over egg noodles, so why not egg*plant* noodles? Turns out that the flavor of the eggplant noodles here pairs wonderfully with the creamy beef. It pays to think outside the box!

SERVES 6

1½ pounds beef sirloin steak, sliced ½ inch thick

Kosher salt and ground black pepper

4 tablespoons salted butter

8 ounces fresh mushrooms, sliced (2½ cups)

1 medium onion, diced

1 clove garlic, chopped

2 cups beef bone broth, homemade (page 35) or store-bought

1 tablespoon Primal-cesterhire Sauce (page 264)

1½ cups full-fat sour cream

Eggplant "Noodles" (recipe follows), for serving

MACRONUTRIENTS PER SERVING
CALORIES: 586
FAT: 36 G/325 CALORIES
CARBOHYDRATE: 11 G/ 44 CALORIES
PROTEIN: 57 G/228 CALORIES

1. Season the steak strips with ½ teaspoon each salt and pepper. In a large skillet, melt 2 tablespoons of the butter over medium-high heat. When the butter starts to foam, add the steak and brown for 2 to 3 minutes per side. Work in batches if needed to avoid crowding the pan. Remove the steak to a bowl and set aside.

2. Reduce the heat to medium. Add the remaining 2 tablespoons butter and add the mushrooms. Sauté the mushrooms until soft, about 5 minutes. Add the onion and garlic, and sauté until the onions start to brown, about 5 minutes more.

3. Pour ½ cup of the beef broth into the skillet and deglaze the pan, using a wooden spoon to scrape any browned bits stuck to the bottom. Stir in the remaining 1½ cups beef broth and the primal-cesterhire sauce. Whisk in 1 cup of the sour cream. Bring the mixture to a boil, then reduce to a simmer. Simmer, stirring occasionally, until the sauce has thickened and the flavors have melded, about 30 minutes.

4. Just before serving, taste the sauce and adjust the salt and pepper. Swirl in the remaining ½ cup of sour cream. Serve over the eggplant "noodles."

EGGPLANT "NOODLES"

SERVES 6

3 to 4 tablespoons avocado oil

1 large eggplant or 4 small Japanese eggplants

¼ teaspoon sea salt

¼ teaspoon ground black pepper

1. Position an oven rack 4 to 6 inches below the broiler. Preheat the broiler to low. Brush a broilerproof baking sheet with ½ tablespoon of the oil.

2. Slice the eggplant crosswise into rounds as thinly as possible, using a mandoline if you have one. Lay the slices on the baking sheet in a single layer. (You will likely need to do this in more than one batch.) Use a pastry brush or oil mister to lightly coat the eggplant with oil, then season with the salt and pepper.

3. Broil the eggplant slices until lightly browned and the edges start to curl slightly. Watch them carefully! Use tongs to transfer them gently to a plate. Allow them to cool slightly. If you used small Japanese eggplants, cut the slices in half. For larger eggplants, cut the slices into 3 to 4 strips.

BRAISED SHORT RIBS WITH MASHED CAULIFLOWER

Short ribs, besides being delicious, are great on a keto diet because they are a fatty cut of meat. As such, they do best with a cooking technique like braising that allows the fat to slowly render. Braising until they are fall-off-the-bone tender is ideal.

SERVES 4

4 large or 8 small bone-in short ribs (about 4 pounds total)

Sea salt and ground black pepper

1 tablespoon lard, bacon fat, or avocado oil

1 small onion, chopped

1 small carrot, chopped

1 stalk celery with leaves, chopped

3 cloves garlic, smashed

2 tablespoons balsamic vinegar

3¼ cups chicken or beef bone broth, homemade (page 35) or store-bought

6 sprigs fresh thyme

1 large head cauliflower, cut into florets

1. Preheat the oven to 325°F.

2. Pat the short ribs dry, then generously season on all sides with salt and pepper.

3. In a cast-iron Dutch oven (see Note) or other ovenproof pan with a lid, heat the lard over medium-high heat. When it starts to smoke, place the short ribs in it in a single layer. Brown until a nice brown crust forms on the outside, 2 to 3 minutes per side. Transfer the short ribs to a plate. Spoon out about 2 tablespoons of fat from the pan and set aside.

4. Reduce the heat to medium under the pan. Add the onion, carrot, celery, and garlic and cook, stirring frequently, until the vegetables start to soften, about 5 minutes. Add the balsamic vinegar and ½ cup of the broth. Deglaze the bottom of the pan, using a wooden spoon to scrape up any browned bits stuck to the bottom. Cook to slightly thicken the sauce, another 2 to 3 minutes.

5. Return the short ribs to the pan along with any accumulated juices. Pour in another 2 cups broth. The short ribs should be mostly covered with liquid. If not, add a bit of water. Nestle the thyme around the short ribs. Allow the liquid to come to a boil. Cover the pan and transfer it to the oven. Set a timer for 1 hour.

recipe continues

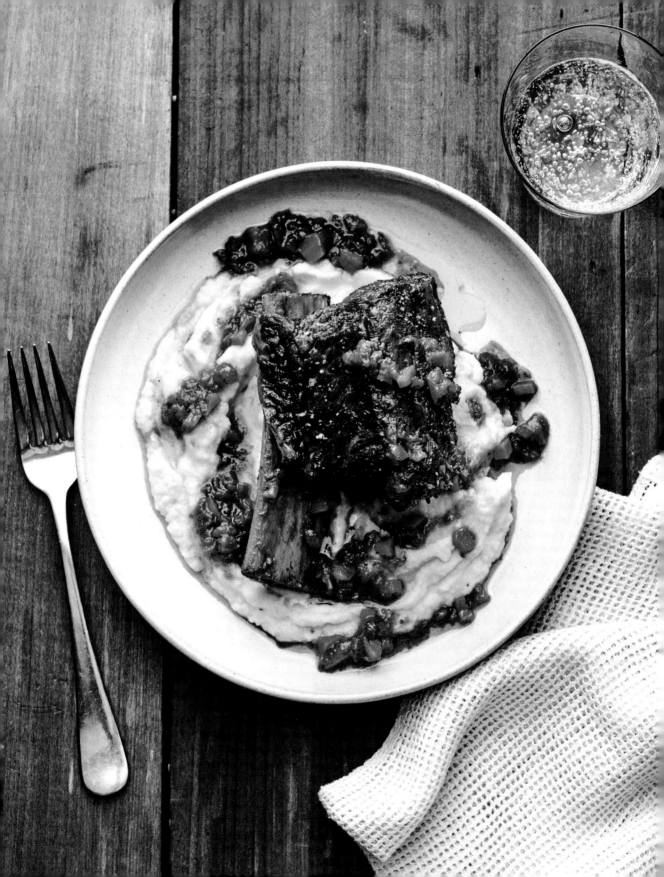

1 tablespoon salted butter,
cut into pieces (optional)

¼ cup fresh parsley leaves,
chopped, for garnish

MACRONUTRIENTS PER SERVING (WITH BUTTER)
CALORIES: 612
FAT: 48 G/432 CALORIES
CARBOHYDRATE: 17 G/ 70 CALORIES
PROTEIN: 29 G/116 CALORIES

Note: If you do not have a Dutch oven, you can use an ovenproof skillet and cover it tightly with foil. Or, use any skillet for steps 3 through 5, then carefully transfer the short ribs, vegetables, and hot braising liquid to a separate covered casserole dish before placing it in the oven.

6. Meanwhile, use the reserved fat to brush the inside of a covered casserole dish large enough to just fit the cauliflower. Add the cauliflower florets and season with ½ teaspoon salt and ¼ teaspoon pepper. Pour the remaining ¾ cup broth into the dish. Place the butter (if using) on top of the cauliflower and cover the casserole dish.

7. When the timer goes off, uncover the short ribs (watch out for steam!), rotate the pan in the oven, and place the cauliflower in the oven with the short ribs. Cook the short ribs for another 1 hour, covered.

8. After the ribs have baked for 2 hours, carefully flip them and cook until the meat is very tender, 45 minutes to 1 hour longer. Check the level of the liquid occasionally. If it reduces by more than about half, add a bit of water.

9. Remove the short ribs and cauliflower from the oven. Carefully ladle as much liquid as you can from the short rib pan (or use a turkey baster), and strain it into a small sauce-pan. Bring the liquid to a boil, then reduce to a simmer until thickened slightly.

10. Transfer the cauliflower to a food processor. Fish the garlic cloves out of the short rib pan (it's okay if they are falling apart, just do your best) and add them to the food processor as well. Process the cauliflower until creamy. Taste and adjust the salt and pepper.

11. To serve, spoon an even portion of the cauliflower mash onto each plate. Place one or two short ribs on top. Top with a few tablespoons of the pan juice. Sprinkle with parsley. Serve hot.

OFFAL BACON BURGERS

These burgers are offal but also awesome! Don't skip the steps of precooking the bacon and liver, or else you'll end up with raw bacon in the middle of your burgers—not the most appealing culinary experience.

SERVES 6

4 slices sugar-free bacon

6 ounces liver (beef or pork), cubed

1¼ pounds ground beef (or a mixture of ground beef and ground beef heart)

¼ cup finely chopped onion

2 cloves garlic, minced

½ teaspoon dried oregano

½ teaspoon dried parsley

¾ teaspoon sea salt

½ teaspoon ground black pepper

FOR SERVING

6 collard green leaves, ribs removed

6 tablespoons avocado oil mayonnaise

2 small avocados, sliced

MACRONUTRIENTS PER SERVING

CALORIES: 550

FAT: 41 G/369 CALORIES

CARBOHYDRATE: 7 G/ 28 CALORIES

PROTEIN: 40 G/160 CALORIES

1. Heat a large skillet over medium heat. Add the bacon and cook until crispy, flipping as needed. Remove the bacon to a plate (leave the fat in the pan).

2. Add the liver to the same pan and cook in the bacon fat until just cooked, about 2 minutes per side. Use a slotted spoon to transfer the liver to a food processor. Crumble the bacon into the food processor and pulse until the meats are finely chopped. Transfer the liver and bacon to a large bowl.

3. Crumble the ground beef into the bowl. Add the onion, garlic, oregano, and parsley. Stir very well until the bacon, liver, and beef are thoroughly incorporated.

4. Form the mixture into 6 patties. Season all over with the salt and pepper. In the same skillet, cook the burgers about 5 minutes per side, or until done to your preference. (Alternatively you can cook these on a grill.)

5. To serve, place each patty on a collard green. Top with 1 tablespoon mayo and some sliced avocado. Wrap the collard green around the patty and secure with a toothpick if desired.

JERK CHICKEN DRUMSTICKS WITH COOLING YOGURT SAUCE

Why are drumsticks fun to eat? You can make the yogurt sauce up to a day ahead; just give it a stir before serving. Pair with Triple-Coconut Cauliflower Rice (page 165).

SERVES 6

¼ cup avocado oil

1 tablespoon Jerk Seasoning Blend (page 254)

Grated zest and juice of ½ lemon

½ teaspoon kosher salt

6 chicken drumsticks

FOR THE YOGURT SAUCE

¾ cup plain full-fat Greek yogurt (or coconut milk or cashew yogurt if dairy-free)

Grated zest and juice of ½ lemon

2 tablespoons fresh cilantro leaves, finely chopped

1 clove garlic, pressed

¼ teaspoon dried thyme

¼ teaspoon sea salt

⅛ teaspoon ground black pepper

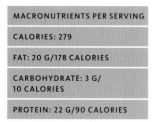

MACRONUTRIENTS PER SERVING

CALORIES: 279

FAT: 20 G/178 CALORIES

CARBOHYDRATE: 3 G/ 10 CALORIES

PROTEIN: 22 G/90 CALORIES

1. In a bowl, mix together the avocado oil, jerk seasoning, lemon zest, lemon juice, and salt. Place the drumsticks in a glass container that will hold them snugly. Pour the oil mixture over them. Shake gently to coat the drumsticks with the marinade, then refrigerate. Marinate for at least 30 minutes but up to 8 hours (longer is better).

2. When you are ready to cook, remove the chicken from the fridge and let stand at room temperature for 15 minutes. Preheat the oven to 425°F.

3. Arrange the chicken in a single layer in a baking dish. Pour any remaining marinade over the chicken. Place the chicken in the oven and set a timer for 20 minutes.

4. Meanwhile, make the yogurt sauce: In a small bowl, mix together the yogurt, lemon zest, lemon juice, cilantro, garlic, thyme, salt, and pepper. (*Optional, but recommended:* Use an immersion blender to blitz the yogurt sauce a few times to make it a little smoother.) Refrigerate the yogurt sauce until serving time.

5. When the timer goes off, flip the drumsticks and bake until the internal temperature reaches 165°F, 15 to 20 minutes longer.

6. Remove the chicken from the oven and let it rest for 5 to 10 minutes before serving. Serve each drumstick with a dollop of the yogurt sauce on top or in a small ramekin for dipping.

TUNA CAKES

This recipe is a nice way to make basic canned tuna more interesting. Serve it with Tartar Sauce (page 263), Aioli (page 262), or the World's Easiest Dipping Sauce (page 183).

SERVES 4

4   (5-ounce) cans albacore tuna (see Note, page 75)

2   large eggs

¾   cup pork rind crumbs (about 0.75 ounce) or ¼ cup almond meal (see Note)

1   small shallot, minced

1   stalk celery, finely chopped

¼   cup olives (green, niçoise, or kalamata), finely chopped

2   tablespoons finely chopped fresh parsley

1   teaspoon fresh lemon juice

½   teaspoon garlic powder

½   teaspoon ground white pepper

¼   teaspoon kosher salt

    Keto-friendly hot sauce (optional)

2   tablespoons avocado oil

1. Flake the tuna into a medium bowl (make sure to include the oil from the can). Lightly beat the eggs and mix them into the tuna. Add the pork rind crumbs, shallot, celery, olives, parsley, lemon juice, garlic powder, white pepper, salt, and hot sauce (if using) to taste and stir very well to combine. Ideally refrigerate the mixture for 1 hour.

2. Divide the tuna mixture into 8 portions and form them into 8 patties about ¾ inch thick. In a large skillet, heat the oil over medium to medium-high heat. Add 4 tuna cakes and cook until crispy on both sides, about 3 minutes per side. Repeat with the remaining 4 cakes, adding more oil if needed. Serve warm or chilled.

Note: You can purchase pork rind crumbs at most grocery stores, or you can grind chicharrones in a small food processor until they reach the consistency of bread crumbs.

Mix it up! Substitute 1 or 2 cans of sardines for the equivalent amount of tuna. You can also use this same recipe to make salmon cakes by swapping out the tuna for an equivalent amount of canned or leftover cooked salmon.

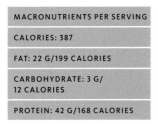

MACRONUTRIENTS PER SERVING

CALORIES: 387

FAT: 22 G/199 CALORIES

CARBOHYDRATE: 3 G/ 12 CALORIES

PROTEIN: 42 G/168 CALORIES

LEMONY BAKED CHICKEN

Baked chicken is a dish that everyone should have in their arsenal. It is both simple and delicious, especially when it involves salty, crispy chicken skin. A lemony pan sauce takes this chicken recipe over the top. For a complete meal, pair this with Buttery Green Beans Amandine (page 174).

SERVES 6

4   bone-in, skin-on chicken breasts

Kosher salt

3   lemons

2   cups + about ½ cup chicken bone broth, homemade (page 35) or store-bought

¾   teaspoon dried rosemary

½   teaspoon dried oregano

¼   teaspoon garlic powder

¼   teaspoon ground black pepper

2   tablespoons butter or ghee, melted

2   egg yolks

MACRONUTRIENTS PER SERVING

CALORIES: 354

FAT: 19 G/171 CALORIES

CARBOHYDRATE: 5 G/ 20 CALORIES

PROTEIN: 40 G/160 CALORIES

1. Take the chicken breasts out of the refrigerator 30 minutes before you want to bake them. Sprinkle liberally with salt.

2. Preheat the oven to 400°F.

3. Grate the zest of one of the lemons and juice all three. Set the zest and juice aside. Place the spent lemon rinds in the baking dish that you will use to bake the chicken. Pour 2 cups of the chicken broth into the baking dish.

4. In a small bowl, mix together the rosemary, oregano, garlic powder, and pepper. Place the chicken skin side up in the baking dish on top of the lemons. Pour the melted butter over the top of the chicken and season with the mixed herbs.

5. Bake until the internal temperature of the chicken reaches 165°F, 40 to 50 minutes. Remove the chicken to a plate and loosely cover.

6. Carefully pour the juices from the baking dish into a glass measuring cup. Add enough additional broth to make 1¼ cups liquid. Set a fine-mesh sieve over a medium saucepan and strain the liquid into the pan.

7. Set the pan over medium heat. In a small bowl, lightly beat together the egg yolks and reserved lemon juice. Slowly whisk the egg yolk mixture into the broth. Cook, whisking frequently, until the sauce is somewhat thickened, 5 to 7 minutes.

8. To serve, arrange the chicken on a warm serving platter. Pour the sauce over the top or transfer it to a small gravy pitcher and serve alongside the chicken.

PAN-SEARED PORK CHOPS WITH CHIMICHURRI

The secret to making juicy pork chops is to not overcook them. They should be *just* cooked through, with the interior showing just a hint of pink. If the color inside is a uniform beige, you have likely overcooked the meat. This recipe provides a pretty fail-safe method, and is quick to boot.

SERVES 4

4   pork chops, 1 inch thick

1   teaspoon ground cumin

2   teaspoons kosher salt

1   teaspoon ground black pepper

2   tablespoons pork lard or fat of choice

Chimichurri (page 261; see Note)

MACRONUTRIENTS PER SERVING (WITHOUT CHIMICHURRI)

CALORIES: 280

FAT: 20 G/177 CALORIES

CARBOHYDRATE: <1 G/ 2 CALORIES

PROTEIN: 24 G/94 CALORIES

1. Ideally, take the pork chops out of the refrigerator 20 to 30 minutes before you intend to cook them. Rub ⅛ teaspoon cumin into each side of the pork chops. Season with the salt and pepper.

2. Preheat the oven to 400°F.

3. When the oven is almost ready, heat the lard in a large cast-iron skillet over medium-high heat. When it just starts to smoke, swirl the pan to completely coat the bottom with the fat. Place the pork chops in the pan and cook without disturbing for 5 minutes. Flip the pork chops. Cook for 1 minute, then carefully transfer the pan to the oven.

4. After 4 minutes, check the thickest part of the chops with an instant-read thermometer. You are aiming for an internal temperature of 140°F. If needed, return the pork chops to the oven for 2 to 3 minutes and check again.

5. When the pork chops are done, remove them from the oven, transfer to a plate, and let rest for about 5 minutes. To serve, plate the pork chops and drizzle generously with chimichurri.

Note: You will likely not use the entire batch of chimichurri for this recipe. Save the rest for using on cooked eggs or grilled vegetables in a future meal.

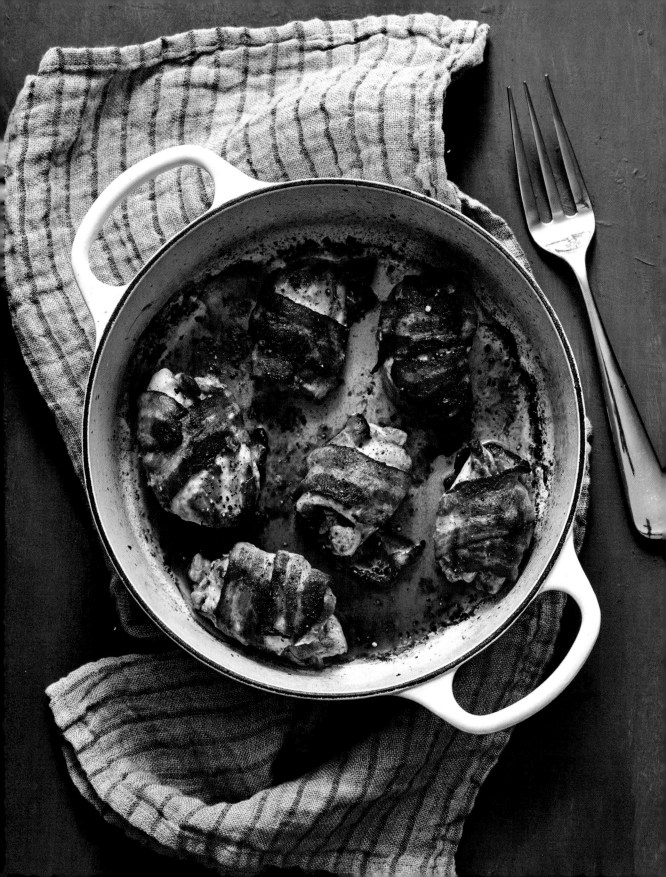

BACON-WRAPPED CHICKEN THIGHS

This is one of those dishes where the whole is greater than the sum of its parts. Bacon and chicken thighs are both delicious, *obviously*, but bacon-wrapped chicken thighs? Fabulous!

SERVES 6

3   tablespoons butter or ghee, melted, or fat of choice

½   teaspoon apple cider vinegar

1   teaspoon mustard powder

½   teaspoon chili powder

¼   teaspoon sea salt

¼   teaspoon ground black pepper

6   boneless, skinless chicken thighs

6   slices sugar-free bacon

MACRONUTRIENTS PER SERVING
CALORIES: 220
FAT: 14 G/122 CALORIES
CARBOHYDRATE: ‹1 G/ 1 CALORIE
PROTEIN: 23 G/91 CALORIES

1. In a medium bowl, combine the melted butter, apple cider vinegar, and all the spices. Trim any excess fat from the chicken thighs and add the thighs to the bowl, tossing to coat them with the butter mixture. Allow it to sit for about 20 minutes, tossing once or twice.

2. Preheat the oven to 400°F.

3. Lay out a piece of bacon on a cutting board. Place a chicken thigh at one end of the bacon slice and roll it up so the bacon winds around the chicken, covering as much of the chicken thigh as possible. (Yes, this is a little messy!) Secure the loose end with a toothpick, or tuck the end under the wrapped bacon. Repeat for the rest of the bacon and chicken thighs.

4. Heat a cast-iron or other ovenproof skillet over medium heat. Place the bacon-wrapped chicken thighs in a single layer in the hot skillet. Cook until the bacon is crispy on one side, 3 to 4 minutes. Flip and cook on the second side for an additional 3 to 4 minutes.

5. Transfer the skillet to the oven and roast until the internal temperature of the chicken reaches 165°F, about 10 minutes for smaller thighs or 15 minutes for larger thighs. Remove the chicken from the oven and allow it to rest for a few minutes before serving.

AHI SEAWEED RICE BOWL

While most of us only get seaweed when it's on a sushi roll, integrating seaweed into your diet more often gives you a great source of iodine, an important nutrient in which many adults are deficient. This recipe calls for both wakame and dulse (also an ingredient in the Three from the Sea Salad, page 75), but you could use other seaweeds such as nori; just make sure you avoid seaweed with added vegetable oil.

SERVES 4

8 thin spears asparagus, woody ends cut off, cut on a diagonal into 3 or 4 pieces

FOR THE TUNA

¾ pound sushi-grade ahi tuna, cut into long rectangular portions

½ cup sesame seeds (white, black, or a mixture)

1 to 2 tablespoons kelp flakes (optional)

3 tablespoons avocado oil, for cooking the tuna

FOR THE SEAWEED RICE

2 tablespoons avocado oil

1 shallot, minced

½ cup dried dulse, finely chopped with a knife or kitchen shears

6 cups riced cauliflower

1 teaspoon sea salt

¼ cup dried wakame, soaked according to package directions

1. Bring a large pot of salted water to a boil. Prepare a bowl of ice water. Drop the asparagus into the boiling water and boil for 2 minutes. Use a slotted spoon to remove the asparagus and place it in the ice water.

2. For the tuna: Pat the outside of the tuna dry. Mix together the sesame seeds and kelp flakes (if using) and place on a plate. Press all sides of the tuna into the sesame seeds (or sesame/kelp mixture) to coat. Set the tuna aside. (Save any remaining sesame seeds for garnish.)

3. For the seaweed rice: In a large skillet or wok, heat the avocado oil over medium-high heat. Add the shallot and stir-fry for 1 minute. Add the chopped dulse and stir-fry for another minute. Stir in the cauliflower rice and salt and stir-fry for 2 minutes. Add the soaked wakame and cook until the cauliflower is tender but not mushy, another 2 to 4 minutes. Remove from the heat.

4. To cook the tuna: In a skillet, heat the avocado oil over medium-high heat. When the oil begins to smoke, carefully place the tuna in the pan. Sear for 45 seconds per side. Remove it to a cutting board and cut the tuna into slices ¼ inch thick.

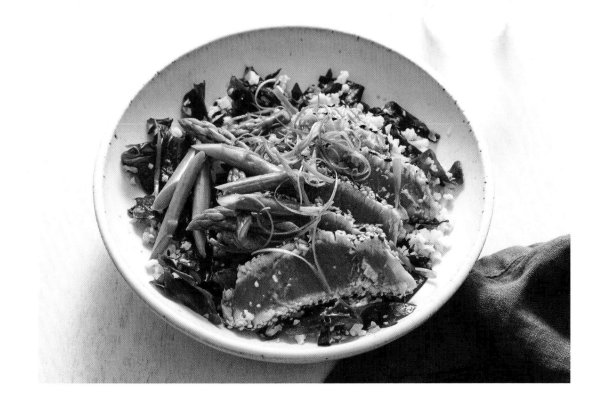

5. For the sauce: In a bowl, whisk together the sesame oil, coconut aminos, vinegar, and ginger.

6. Divide the cauliflower rice among four bowls. Top each with equal portions of the sliced tuna. Drain the asparagus, pat dry, and distribute evenly among the four bowls. Drizzle the sauce over the tuna. Sprinkle with the scallions and any remaining sesame seeds from step 2.

Note: The sesame seeds add 4 grams of carbohydrate per serving in this recipe. If you want to omit them to save the carbs, simply season the ahi with the kelp flakes, salt, and pepper.

FOR THE SAUCE AND GARNISH

- 2 tablespoons sesame oil
- 2 tablespoons coconut aminos or tamari
- 1 tablespoon coconut vinegar or vinegar of choice

   1-inch piece fresh ginger, peeled and very finely grated
- 2 scallions, finely chopped, for garnish

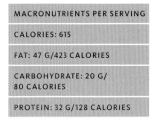

MACRONUTRIENTS PER SERVING
CALORIES: 615
FAT: 47 G/423 CALORIES
CARBOHYDRATE: 20 G/ 80 CALORIES
PROTEIN: 32 G/128 CALORIES

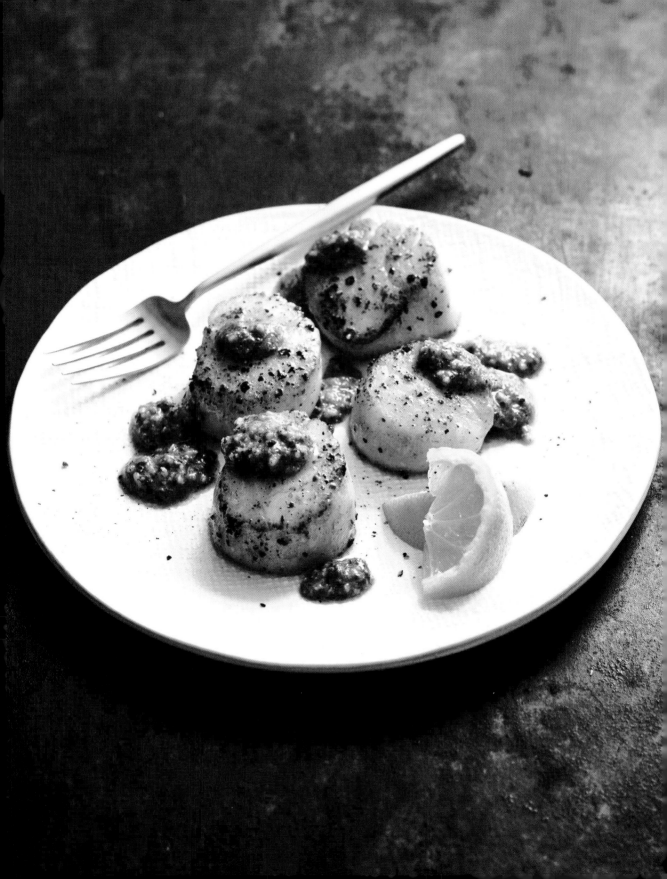

BRAD'S SCALLOPS WITH PESTO

This is the recipe that *The Keto Reset Diet* coauthor, Brad Kearns, serves whenever he wants to impress his dinner guests. Little do they know how simple it actually is. If you use store-bought pesto, this dish comes together in under 5 minutes—just be sure to avoid refined vegetable oils, which often find their way into the mixture.

SERVES 4

16 sea scallops (about 20 ounces)

1 teaspoon kosher salt

½ teaspoon ground black pepper

1 tablespoon unsalted butter

1 tablespoon avocado oil

½ cup pesto, homemade (page 265) or store-bought

1 lemon, cut into wedges

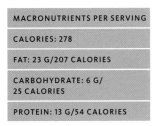

MACRONUTRIENTS PER SERVING

CALORIES: 278

FAT: 23 G/207 CALORIES

CARBOHYDRATE: 6 G/ 25 CALORIES

PROTEIN: 13 G/54 CALORIES

1. Rinse the scallops and pat them dry. Line a plate with a clean kitchen towel and place the scallops on it to dry further. Season the tops and bottoms with the salt and pepper.

2. In a large skillet, heat the butter and avocado oil over medium heat. When the oil is hot, place the scallops in a single layer in the pan so they are not touching. Cook for 90 seconds without disturbing. Flip the scallops and cook another 90 seconds on the second side (2 minutes if they are quite large). The scallops should still be *just* translucent in the middle. If they are cooked to the point of being rubbery and with white interiors, they are overcooked. If you're a little nervous that you undercooked them, you probably nailed it!

3. Divide the scallops among four serving plates. Top each scallop with a generous dollop of pesto and serve with a lemon wedge.

CRISPY BAKED COD WITH TARTAR SAUCE

The fact is, no keto-friendly option can match a traditional battered and fried fish fillet, but this version packs both flavor and crunch thanks to a pork rind "crust."

SERVES 4

4 cod fillets (about 4 ounces each)

½ teaspoon sea salt

¼ teaspoon ground black pepper

⅓ cup pork rind crumbs (see Note)

2 tablespoons grated Parmesan cheese (see Note)

1 tablespoon Cajun Seasoning (page 253)

3 tablespoons avocado oil mayonnaise

1 lemon, cut into wedges

Tartar Sauce (page 263)

MACRONUTRIENTS PER SERVING
CALORIES: 490
FAT: 43 G/391 CALORIES
CARBOHYDRATE: 3 G/ 13 CALORIES
PROTEIN: 21 G/86 CALORIES

1. Preheat the oven to 400°F.

2. Pat the cod dry, then season both sides with the salt and pepper. In a small food processor, combine the pork rind crumbs, Parmesan, and Cajun seasoning and pulse a few times to combine. Brush or spread about 1 teaspoon mayo on the top of each piece of fish. Press 1 tablespoon of the pork rind mixture into the mayo. Gently flip the fish and repeat on the other side.

3. Set a wire rack in a rimmed baking sheet. Gently transfer the fish to the wire rack, being careful not to knock off the pork rinds. Bake until the fish is firm, about 15 minutes. (*Optional:* Heat the broiler to low and place the fish under the broiler for 1 minute to crisp up the "breading.")

4. Remove the fish from the oven and use a spatula to carefully transfer it to serving plates. Serve with lemon wedges and individual ramekins of tartar sauce.

Note: If you avoid dairy, omit the Parmesan cheese and increase the pork rind crumbs to ½ cup.

Mix it up!
- Have a hankering for fish and chips? Serve this fish with the daikon radish fries from Keto Poutine (page 184) or the Jícama Fries (page 182)!
- For a fun twist, make your tartar sauce with Primal Kitchen Chipotle Lime Mayo (see Note, page 183). Keep all the other ingredients the same, but omit the hot sauce.

PARMESAN POPCORN SHRIMP

Warning: These little shrimp are highly addictive. In the oven, as the Parmesan melts, the saltiness of the cheese intensifies and mixes with the spices. You should probably just go ahead and double or triple the recipe to start—it's going to disappear that fast.

SERVES 4

1   pound small shrimp, peeled and deveined

5   tablespoons butter or ghee, melted

2   teaspoons fresh lemon juice, at room temperature

2   cups finely grated Parmesan cheese

¼   cup fresh parsley leaves, finely chopped

1   teaspoon smoked paprika

1   teaspoon garlic powder

1   teaspoon ground white pepper

½   teaspoon celery salt or sea salt

½   teaspoon ground black pepper

1. Preheat the oven to 400°F. Line a rimmed baking sheet with parchment paper.

2. Rinse the shrimp and pat dry with a clean kitchen towel. In a medium bowl, stir together the melted butter and lemon juice. Add the shrimp and toss very well to coat.

3. In a food processor, combine the Parmesan, parsley, paprika, garlic powder, white pepper, celery salt, and black pepper and pulse several times to combine. Transfer the Parmesan mixture to a shallow bowl or small baking dish.

4. Stir the shrimp again. Move a few shrimp at a time to the Parmesan mixture and toss to coat. Press the cheese into the shrimp, then carefully transfer them to the prepared baking sheet. Repeat for the rest of the shrimp. Sprinkle any remaining cheese over the shrimp and pat down.

5. Bake for 10 minutes. Remove from the oven and let sit for a few minutes before serving.

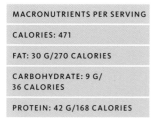

MACRONUTRIENTS PER SERVING

CALORIES: 471

FAT: 30 G/270 CALORIES

CARBOHYDRATE: 9 G/ 36 CALORIES

PROTEIN: 42 G/168 CALORIES

KETO KADDO BOURANI

Kaddo bourani **is an Afghan dish in which spiced ground beef is served over a pile of cubed (sometimes candied) pumpkin and topped with yogurt sauce (see Note). The flavors are outstanding, but the pumpkin-to-meat ratio is a little unbalanced to be keto-friendly. This recipe captures the spirit of the original dish but with a balance that is more consistent with keto macros.**

SERVES 4

FOR THE SAUCE

½ cup full-fat coconut milk

½ cup plain full-fat Greek yogurt, coconut milk yogurt, or kefir

Juice of 1 lemon

1 clove garlic, pressed or finely minced

¼ cup fresh mint leaves, very finely chopped

MACRONUTRIENTS PER SERVING

CALORIES: 621

FAT: 41 G/366 CALORIES

CARBOHYDRATE: 14 G/ 56 CALORIES

PROTEIN: 48 G/190 CALORIES

---

1. For the sauce: In a small bowl, combine the coconut milk, yogurt, lemon juice, garlic, and mint. Place in the refrigerator to chill.

2. For the beef mixture: In a large skillet, heat the avocado oil over medium heat. Add the onion and garlic and sauté until the onion is translucent, about 4 minutes. Crumble in the ground beef and cook until browned through, breaking up the meat as it cooks, 8 to 10 minutes.

3. In a small bowl, mix together all the spices and sprinkle the mixture over the meat. Stir well to combine, then cook for 2 minutes. Stir in the tomatoes and water. Increase the heat to medium-high and bring the liquid to a boil, then reduce the heat to a simmer. Simmer uncovered until the liquid has mostly evaporated, about 15 minutes. Meanwhile, heat the pumpkin puree in a small saucepan over medium-low heat until warm, 4 to 5 minutes.

4. Divide the meat among four serving bowls and top each with ¼ cup pumpkin puree. Serve with the yogurt sauce poured over the top.

Note: This dish is also great served over a bed of zucchini noodles or spaghetti squash. If you want to omit the pumpkin, it won't be *kaddo bourani* anymore, but the meat mixture still makes a wonderful topping for veggie noodles or Basic Cauliflower Rice (page 37).

- 1 tablespoon avocado oil or fat of choice
- 1 small onion, chopped
- 2 cloves garlic, chopped
- 1½ pounds ground beef
- 1½ teaspoons kosher salt
- 1 teaspoon ground black pepper
- 1 teaspoon ground turmeric
- ¾ teaspoon ground coriander
- ½ teaspoon ground ginger
- ¼ teaspoon ground cinnamon
- ¼ teaspoon red pepper flakes (optional)
- 2 small tomatoes, seeded and chopped
- 1 cup filtered water or beef bone broth, homemade (page 35) or store-bought
- 1 cup Homemade Pumpkin Puree (page 245) or unsweetened canned

SHEPHERD'S PIE

Shepherd's pie is total comfort food. It usually involves ground meat (beef or lamb) mixed with peas and topped with mashed potatoes. Obviously it needs some adjusting to be made primal- and keto-friendly, but that is easy to do. Make sure you don't skimp on the mashed cauliflower topping in this recipe—you want a nice thick "crust."

SERVES 6

2 medium heads cauliflower, cut into florets (about 8 cups)

1 small parsnip, peeled and cubed (see Note)

6 slices sugar-free bacon, chopped

1 small onion, chopped

3 stalks celery with leaves, chopped

1 small carrot, chopped

1½ pounds ground beef (or half ground pork or ground lamb)

½ teaspoon dried thyme

   Kosher salt and ground black pepper

1 cup chicken or beef bone broth, homemade (page 35) or store-bought

2 tablespoons Primal-cestershire Sauce (page 264)

2 tablespoons butter

1. Preheat the oven to 400°F.

2. In a large pot fitted with a steamer basket, bring 1 to 2 inches of water to a boil. Place the cauliflower and parsnip in the steamer, cover, and steam until the vegetables can be easily pierced with a fork, about 15 minutes.

3. Meanwhile, heat a large skillet over medium heat. Cook the bacon until crispy, then transfer to a plate and set aside.

4. Add the onion, celery, and carrot to the bacon fat in the pan and sauté until the vegetables are soft, about 5 minutes. Crumble in the ground meat and season with the thyme, ½ teaspoon salt, and ¼ teaspoon pepper. Cook, breaking up the meat with a fork or meat chopper, until only a little pink remains, about 5 minutes.

5. Crumble the cooked bacon into the ground meat mixture. Stir in the broth and primal-cestershire sauce and cook until the broth has reduced by about half, another 8 to 10 minutes. Continue to break up the meat as it simmers.

6. Meanwhile, place the cooked cauliflower and parsnips in a food processor with the butter and ¼ teaspoon each salt and pepper. Process until smooth. You might need to do this in batches, in which case divide the butter between the batches. Transfer the mashed cauliflower and parsnips to a large bowl and stir well. Mix in the sour cream (if using). Taste and adjust the salt and pepper.

7. Transfer the meat mixture to a 11.5 × 7-inch or a large oval baking dish. Spoon the cauliflower mash over the top and smooth it with a spatula. (*Optional:* Brush the beaten egg over the top of the cauliflower mash and sprinkle with the Parmesan.) Bake until the mixture is bubbling and the cauliflower is browned, 20 to 30 minutes. Remove from the oven and let rest for 5 minutes before serving.

Note: You might think you have to avoid parsnips on a keto diet since they are a higher-carb root vegetable, but a small parsnip only adds about 1 gram of carbohydrate per serving. However, feel free to omit it if you wish.

¼ cup full-fat sour cream (optional)

1 egg, beaten (optional)

¾ cup grated Parmesan cheese (optional)

MACRONUTRIENTS PER SERVING (WITH ALL OPTIONAL INGREDIENTS)
CALORIES: 516
FAT: 32 G/288 CALORIES
CARBOHYDRATE: 17 G/ 68 CALORIES
PROTEIN: 41 G/164 CALORIES

VEGGIES & SIDES

GARLICKY MUSHROOMS

Looking for a way to dress up your steak dinner? Look no further.

4 tablespoons unsalted butter or fat of choice

6 cups white button mushrooms (about 20 ounces), quartered

4 large cloves garlic, minced

2 tablespoons dry red wine or balsamic vinegar

1 tablespoon fresh oregano leaves

1 teaspoon sea salt

MACRONUTRIENTS PER SERVING

CALORIES: 145

FAT: 12 G/108 CALORIES

CARBOHYDRATE: 6 G/ 24 CALORIES

PROTEIN: 5 G/19 CALORIES

1. In a large skillet, melt the butter over medium heat. Add the mushrooms and sauté, stirring occasionally, until they are soft, about 10 minutes.

2. Push the mushrooms to the edge of the pan. In the cleared space, add the garlic and sauté, stirring frequently, until fragrant, about 1 minute.

3. Stir the mushrooms and garlic together. Stir in the wine, oregano, and salt.

4. Reduce the heat to low and cook, stirring occasionally, until the wine has reduced, about 10 minutes more. Serve warm or at room temperature.

TRIPLE-COCONUT CAULIFLOWER RICE

If you think cauliflower rice is bland and boring, you must try this recipe! Coconut is the perfect complement to add some pizazz to this keto meal staple.

SERVES 4

- 2 tablespoons coconut oil
- 1 pound riced cauliflower (store-bought or from 1 medium head)
- ½ cup coconut cream (see Note, page 229)
- ½ teaspoon sea salt
- ¼ cup unsweetened coconut flakes
- ¼ teaspoon ground cinnamon

MACRONUTRIENTS PER SERVING

CALORIES: 279

FAT: 24 G/216 CALORIES

CARBOHYDRATE: 15 G/ 60 CALORIES

PROTEIN: 6 G/24 CALORIES

1. In a large, deep skillet, heat the coconut oil over medium-high heat. When hot, add the riced cauliflower and stir to coat it with the oil. Spread the rice evenly in the pan and cook without stirring for 3 minutes.

2. Stir the cauliflower rice. Stir in the coconut cream and salt. Cook another 3 to 5 minutes, stirring occasionally. Taste the rice to test the texture. If it is not done to your liking, cook another 1 to 2 minutes and test again. When it reaches the desired texture, transfer the cauliflower rice to a serving bowl.

3. Heat a small skillet over medium heat for 1 minute. Reduce the heat to medium-low and add the coconut flakes and cinnamon. Cook, stirring constantly, until the coconut is lightly toasted, about 1 minute. Sprinkle the coconut flakes over the coconut rice. Serve hot.

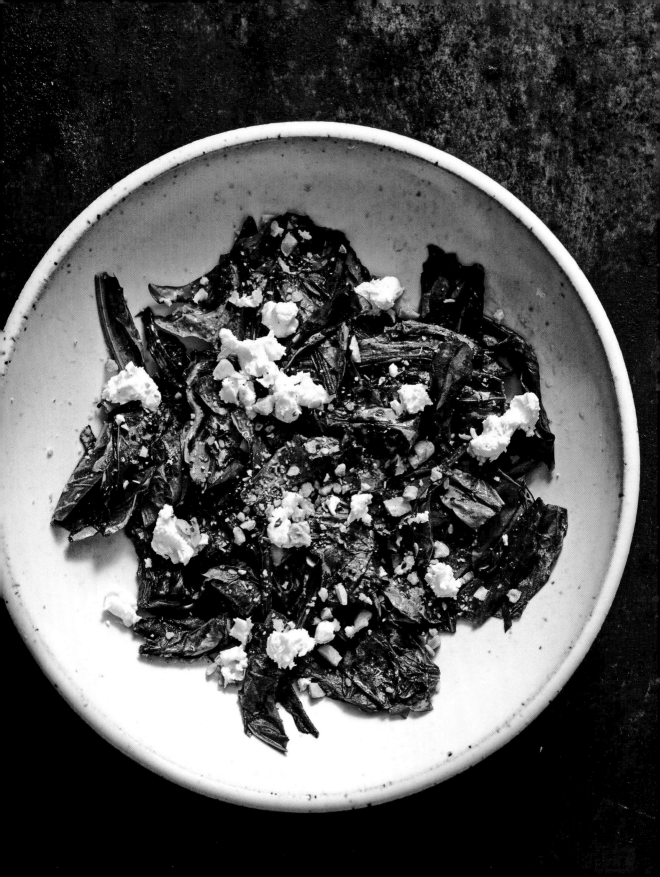

CRISPY DANDELION GREENS WITH HAZELNUTS

Don't skip the blanching step in this recipe. It cuts down the bitterness of the greens and really makes a difference in the final dish. Omit the goat cheese if you are dairy-free.

SERVES 4

- 2   large bunches dandelion greens
- 2   teaspoons ghee
- 1   large clove garlic, minced
- ¼   teaspoon kosher salt
- 1   tablespoon Za'atar Seasoning (page 255; see Note)
- ½   cup crumbled goat cheese
- ¼   cup hazelnuts
- ½   teaspoon extra-virgin olive oil

MACRONUTRIENTS PER SERVING

CALORIES: 140

FAT: 11 G/96 CALORIES

CARBOHYDRATE: 7 G/ 28 CALORIES

PROTEIN: 6 G/24 CALORIES

1. Wash the dandelion greens thoroughly. Trim the ends from the stems and roughly chop the leaves into 2-inch pieces.

2. Bring a large pot of salted water to a boil. Blanch the leaves for 10 minutes. Drain thoroughly in a sieve or colander, then pat them dry with a clean kitchen towel. Separate any clumps of leaves that are stuck together.

3. In a skillet, melt the ghee over medium heat. Add the garlic and dandelion greens and sprinkle with the salt and za'atar. Sauté until the edges of the greens become crispy, about 3 minutes.

4. Divide the sautéed greens among four plates. Sprinkle with the goat cheese. Use a nut grinder or food processor to crush the hazelnuts, and sprinkle them over the goat cheese. Drizzle with a little olive oil and serve warm or at room temperature.

Note: Za'atar is a delicious and versatile seasoning blend, well worth having on hand for a variety of dishes, such as Creamy Za'atar Slaw (page 179). However, you can substitute 1¼ teaspoons dried thyme, 1¼ teaspoons ground cumin, and ½ teaspoon kosher salt in step 3. Finish the salad with a squeeze of fresh lemon juice.

ITALIAN STUFFED SPAGHETTI SQUASH

Stuffed spaghetti squash is a dish your whole family will enjoy. What's not to love about a vegetable that's also its own serving bowl? It is easy enough for a weeknight meal, and tasty and attractive enough that you would also happily serve it at your next dinner party.

SERVES 8

1 medium spaghetti squash

1 tablespoon avocado oil

1½ teaspoons kosher salt

Ground black pepper

1 medium tomato, diced

½ cup loosely packed fresh basil leaves, finely chopped

¼ cup loosely packed fresh parsley leaves, finely chopped

3 cloves garlic, minced

1 (8-ounce) log or ball fresh mozzarella cheese

¾ cup whole-milk ricotta cheese

MACRONUTRIENTS PER SERVING

CALORIES: 325

FAT: 24 G/213 CALORIES

CARBOHYDRATE: 11 G/ 42 CALORIES

PROTEIN: 19 G/75 CALORIES

1. Preheat the oven to 425°F.

2. Use a sharp knife to score the spaghetti squash lengthwise from the stem end down to the blossom end and then back up the other side to the stem end again: This is where you will cut it in half in the next step. Microwave the whole thing on high for 5 minutes.

3. Carefully cut the spaghetti squash in half (it will be hot!). Scoop out and discard the seeds. Brush the inside of the spaghetti squash with the avocado oil and sprinkle with ½ teaspoon each salt and pepper.

4. Place the spaghetti squash cut side down in a glass baking dish. Bake until a knife easily pierces the skin, about 30 minutes.

5. Meanwhile, in a large bowl, stir together the tomato, basil, parsley, garlic, ½ teaspoon pepper, and the remaining 1 teaspoon salt. Divide the mozzarella in half. Cut half the mozzarella into ½-inch cubes and add it to the bowl with the tomatoes and herbs. Thinly slice the other half of the mozzarella and set aside.

6. Remove the spaghetti squash from the oven (but leave the oven on). Use a fork to carefully scoop the strands of the spaghetti squash from the shell, being careful not to tear the shell. (Use a clean kitchen towel to hold the squash so you do

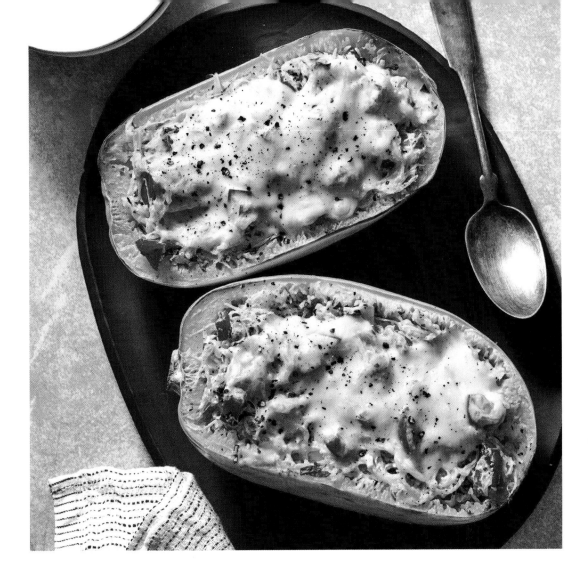

Mix it up! Add 2 cups (10 ounces) cubed cooked chicken or cooked Italian sausage to the mixture in step 5 to make it a complete meal!

not burn your hand.) Add the spaghetti squash "noodles" to the bowl with the tomatoes. Add the ricotta cheese and stir very well to combine.

7. Return the empty spaghetti squash shells cut side up to the baking dish. Spoon the noodle mixture back into the shells. Top with the sliced mozzarella and additional pepper. Return the dish to the oven to melt the cheese, about 15 minutes. (*Optional:* Heat the broiler to low and place the squash under the broiler for a minute to brown the cheese.) Remove the dish from the oven and serve hot.

GARLICKY ROASTED BROCCOLI

If you are not a fan of broccoli, it might be because you only know boring, mushy steamed broccoli. Roasted broccoli is infinitely better than its sad cousin. Throw a little garlic in there (or a lot of garlic!), and you have a real winner.

SERVES 4

4   cloves garlic, pressed or finely minced

2   tablespoons salted butter or ghee, melted

2   tablespoons avocado oil

6   cups broccoli florets (about 14 ounces)

Generous pinch of kosher salt

MACRONUTRIENTS PER SERVING

CALORIES: 150

FAT: 13 G/117 CALORIES

CARBOHYDRATE: 8 G/ 32 CALORIES

PROTEIN: 3 G/12 CALORIES

1. Preheat the oven to 425°F.

2. In a large bowl, stir together the garlic, melted butter, and avocado oil. Add the broccoli and toss very well to completely coat the broccoli.

3. Transfer the broccoli to a heavy rimmed baking sheet. Use a spatula to scrape any remaining butter and garlic from the bowl over the broccoli. Spread the broccoli evenly on the baking sheet and sprinkle with the salt.

4. Roast for 10 minutes. Remove and stir the broccoli. Spread it back out on the pan and return it to the oven to roast another 5 minutes. It is done when the edges of the florets start to brown and crisp. Transfer to a serving bowl and serve hot or at room temperature.

STICKY
BRUSSELS SPROUTS

You might just want to go ahead and double this recipe now, because you will be sad when these are gone!

1   pound Brussels sprouts

2   tablespoons bacon fat or fat of choice

¼   cup balsamic vinaigrette

½   cup full-fat coconut milk

     Sea salt

MACRONUTRIENTS PER SERVING*
CALORIES: 170
FAT: 13 G/117 CALORIES
CARBOHYDRATE: 12 G/ 48 CALORIES
PROTEIN: 6 G/24 CALORIES
* Macros based on using Primal Kitchen Balsamic Vinaigrette.

1. Trim the ends off the Brussels sprouts and remove any damaged outer leaves. Cut the Brussels sprouts in half.

2. In a large skillet or wok with a tight-fitting lid, heat the bacon fat over medium heat. Add the Brussels sprouts to the hot pan and stir to coat with the fat. Cover and cook for 5 minutes, stirring once.

3. Add the balsamic vinaigrette and stir to coat the sprouts. Cover the pan and cook for 2 minutes. Uncover and stir. Pour in the coconut milk, use a wooden spoon to scrape the bottom of the pan, and stir again. Cover and cook 2 more minutes.

4. Remove the lid and test one of the Brussels sprouts. If it is not done to your preference, cover and cook 2 minutes more. Salt to taste. Serve hot.

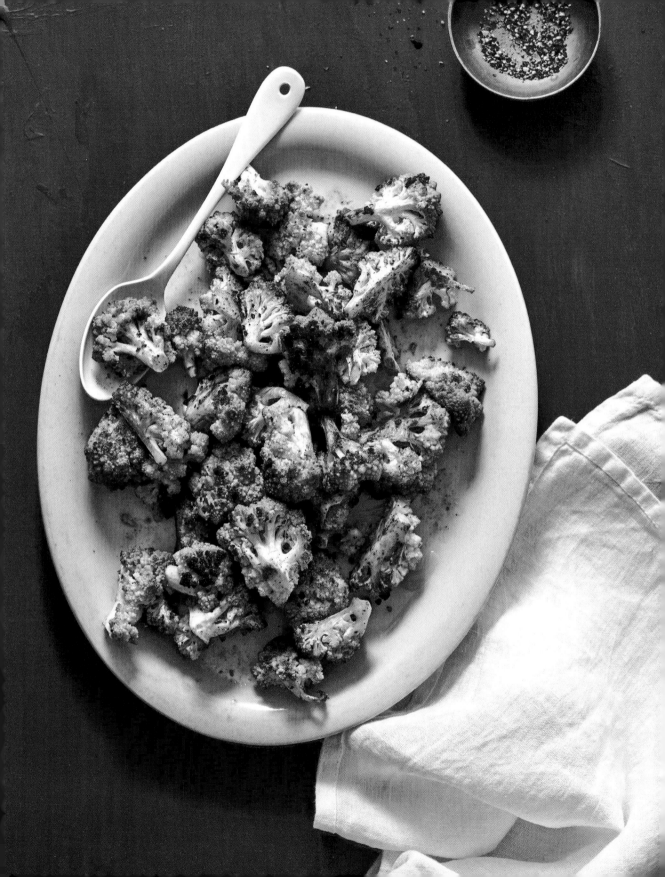

CURRIED ROMANESCO

Lots of readers tell us they tried Romanesco for the first time thanks to the Whole Roasted Romanesco recipe in *The Keto Reset Diet*. Here is another way to use this awesome fractal-icious veggie. Kind of a cross between broccoli and cauliflower, Romanesco is both delicious and beautiful.

SERVES 4

3   tablespoons coconut oil or ghee, melted

1   teaspoon curry powder

½   teaspoon sea salt

2   small heads Romanesco, cut into florets (about 6 cups)

MACRONUTRIENTS PER SERVING
CALORIES: 198
FAT: 17 G/153 CALORIES
CARBOHYDRATE: 6 G/ 24 CALORIES
PROTEIN: 3 G/12 CALORIES

1. Preheat the oven to 425°F.

2. Place the coconut oil in a large bowl and stir in the curry powder and salt. Add the Romanesco florets and toss very well to coat with the spices.

3. Transfer to a large rimmed baking sheet and spread out in a single layer. Roast for 10 minutes. Remove from the oven, stir, and return to the oven for 10 minutes more. It is done when the florets are starting to brown and can be pierced with a fork. Transfer to a serving bowl. Enjoy hot or at room temperature.

BUTTERY GREEN BEANS AMANDINE

How can you go wrong with something described as "buttery"? The flavors of this dish belie how quick and easy it is to make. It pairs well with just about any type of meat, poultry, or seafood.

SERVES 4

6 tablespoons salted butter

1 pound frozen green beans, thawed and drained

Juice of 1 lemon

¼ cup slivered almonds

MACRONUTRIENTS PER SERVING

CALORIES: 234

FAT: 21 G/189 CALORIES

CARBOHYDRATE: 11 G/ 45 CALORIES

PROTEIN: 4 G/15 CALORIES

1. In a large skillet, melt the butter over medium-high heat until it starts to foam. Add the green beans and stir-fry for 3 minutes. Add the lemon juice and stir to combine. Cook until the beans reach desired tenderness, another 1 to 2 minutes. Use tongs to transfer the beans to a serving bowl, but leave some butter in the bottom of the skillet.

2. Reduce the heat under the pan to medium-low, add the almonds, and cook, stirring frequently, until lightly browned, about 2 minutes.

3. Use a spatula to scrape the butter and almonds over the green beans. Toss lightly, then serve immediately.

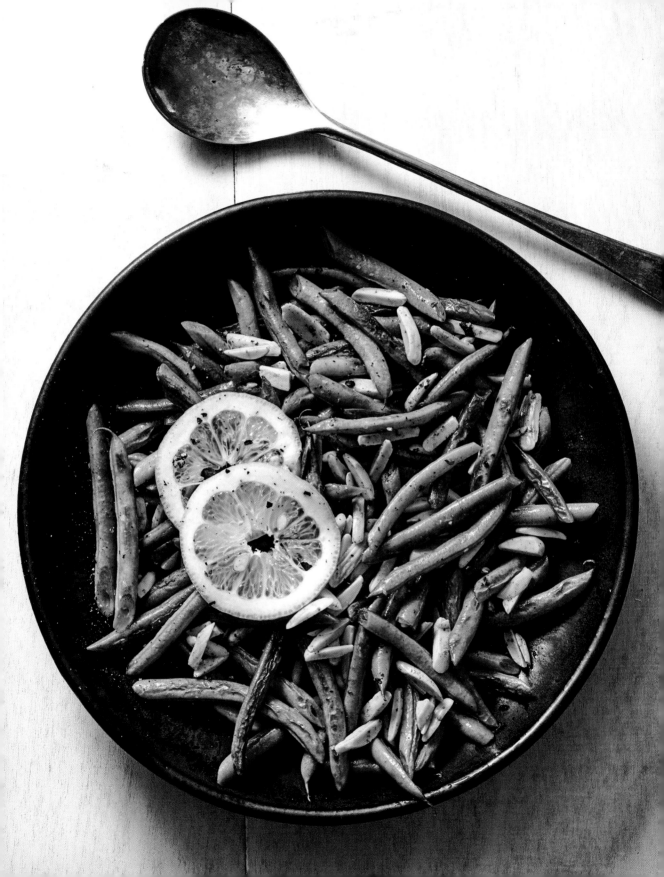

DAIRY-FREE "CHEESY" BROCCOLI

Even if you happily eat cheese, this is still a must-try dish. When you roast the broccoli, the nutritional yeast becomes a cross between a cheese and a crust. It's next-level roasted broccoli for sure! Don't be surprised when you don't have any leftovers.

SERVES 6

1	pound bite-size broccoli florets (about 8 cups)
¼	cup avocado oil
⅓	cup nutritional yeast
1	teaspoon sea salt
½	teaspoon garlic powder
½	teaspoon mustard powder

MACRONUTRIENTS PER SERVING

CALORIES: 142

FAT: 10 G/90 CALORIES

CARBOHYDRATE: 10 G/ 40 CALORIES

PROTEIN: 6 G/24 CALORIES

1. Preheat the oven to 425°F.

2. Place the broccoli in a large bowl and toss very well with the avocado oil.

3. In a small bowl, mix together the nutritional yeast, salt, garlic powder, and mustard powder. Sprinkle half the mixture over the broccoli and toss well. Sprinkle the other half over the broccoli and toss again.

4. Transfer the broccoli to a large, heavy rimmed baking sheet and spread it out in a single layer. Scrape out any nutritional yeast mixture that remains in the bowl and sprinkle it over the broccoli.

5. Roast the broccoli for 10 minutes. Remove it from the oven, stir, spread it out again, and return it to the oven until the broccoli can be pierced with a fork but is still crisp-tender, about 5 minutes more. Transfer the broccoli to a serving bowl and serve hot or at room temperature.

BRAISED RED CABBAGE

If you aim to eat a rainbow assortment of vegetables each day, red cabbage should be a staple. While it's great raw, something special happens when you braise it. Around the 20- to 30-minute mark, a delicate sweetness emerges. If you cut the braising time short, it will still be delicious, but it won't be quite the same.

SERVES 6

- 1 small head red cabbage (1¼ pounds)
- 2 tablespoons bacon fat or fat of choice
- 1 teaspoon caraway seeds
- 2 cloves garlic, chopped

  Sea salt and ground black pepper
- ½ cup chicken or beef bone broth, homemade (page 35) or store-bought, or vegetable stock
- 2 teaspoons apple cider vinegar
- 1 teaspoon Dijon mustard
- 1 teaspoon balsamic vinegar

MACRONUTRIENTS PER SERVING
CALORIES: 77
FAT: 5 G/43 CALORIES
CARBOHYDRATE: 8 G/ 32 CALORIES
PROTEIN: 2 G/8 CALORIES

1. Quarter the cabbage through the core. Use a sharp knife to carefully remove the core. Slice the cabbage into thin strips about ¼ inch thick.

2. In a large high-sided skillet, heat the bacon fat over medium heat. Add the caraway seeds and cook, stirring constantly, for 30 seconds. Add the garlic and cook until soft, about 1 minute. Stir in the shredded cabbage, 1 teaspoon salt, and ½ teaspoon pepper. Allow the cabbage to cook undisturbed for 4 minutes to create some browning. Stir and cook for 4 to 5 minutes more to create some more browning.

3. Meanwhile, in a small bowl, whisk together the broth, apple cider vinegar, mustard, and balsamic vinegar.

4. Toss the cabbage very well in the skillet. Add the broth mixture to the pan and stir well. Reduce the heat to medium-low and cook until the liquid has evaporated and the cabbage is soft but not mushy, 20 to 25 minutes. If the liquid is evaporating too fast, turn the heat down a bit and/or add a couple tablespoons more broth.

5. Taste and adjust the salt and pepper. Serve warm.

TIP: If you're trying to get a bit more fat into your meal, this cabbage is delicious topped with a dollop of sour cream or the horseradish dipping sauce from the Roast Beef Bites (page 206).

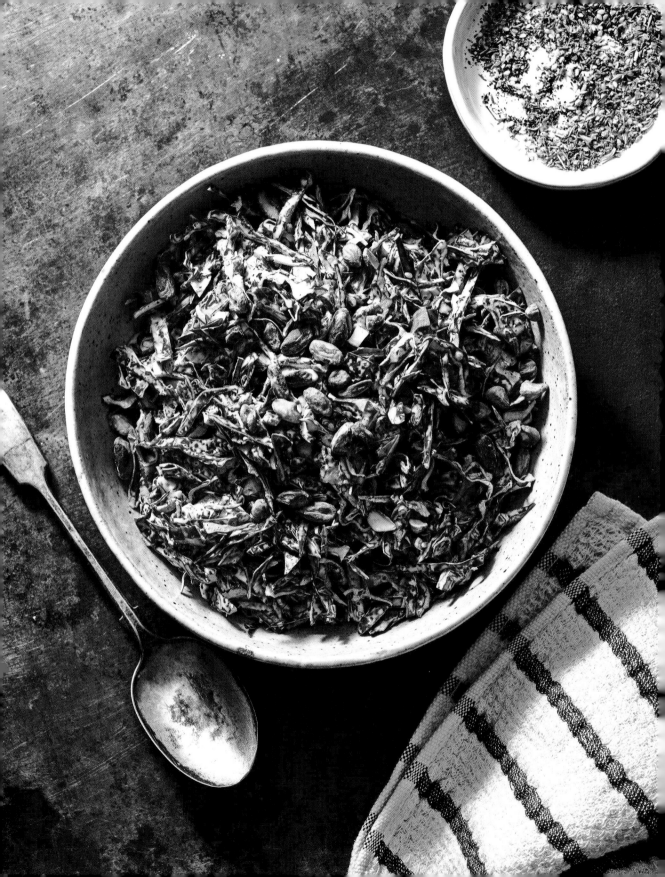

CREAMY ZA'ATAR SLAW (LEBANESE INSPIRED)

If you're not familiar with za'atar, it's time to become acquainted. The main ingredient, sumac, is slightly lemony and distinct without being overpowering. Here, the za'atar adds a special twist to what would otherwise be a basic cabbage slaw.

SERVES 4

⅓ cup full-fat sour cream

2 tablespoons avocado oil mayonnaise

2 teaspoons fresh lemon juice

1 to 2 cloves garlic, minced, or ¼ teaspoon garlic powder

1½ tablespoons Za'atar Seasoning (page 255)

2 tablespoons finely chopped fresh parsley

Sea salt and ground black pepper

4 cups (about 12 ounces) finely shredded red cabbage or other vegetables (see Note)

¼ cup salted roasted pistachios (optional)

1. In a large bowl, mix together the sour cream, mayo, lemon juice, garlic, za'atar, and parsley. Taste and adjust with salt and pepper.

2. Add the shredded cabbage and stir very well to combine. Refrigerate for at least 1 hour.

3. Remove the slaw from the fridge and stir well. Sprinkle with the pistachios (if using) right before serving.

Note: You can use all red cabbage for this recipe or a combination of red and green cabbage. This is also a great way to use up leftover raw broccoli stems (just peel and shred), radishes, kohlrabi, or any other crunchy vegetable you eat raw. If you're in a hurry, bagged slaw mixes from the grocery store work just fine.

MACRONUTRIENTS PER SERVING

CALORIES: 176

FAT: 14 G/126 CALORIES

CARBOHYDRATE: 11 G/ 44 CALORIES

PROTEIN: 4 G/16 CALORIES

FAUX ONION STRAWS

These onion straws (which are more daikon radish than onion) are just what you need for topping your next chicken salad or big juicy steak! They have none of the traditional breading but all of the flavor thanks to two surprise ingredients: hemp and flax.

SERVES 4

1   large purple daikon radish, peeled and ends trimmed (see Note)

½   small onion, sliced as thinly as possible

¼   cup avocado oil

2   tablespoons hemp hearts

2   tablespoons ground flaxseeds

½   teaspoon sea salt

MACRONUTRIENTS PER SERVING
CALORIES: 131
FAT: 11 G/99 CALORIES
CARBOHYDRATE: 6 G/ 24 CALORIES
PROTEIN: 3 G/12 CALORIES

Note: If you can't find purple daikon (they are about the size of a large russet potato, but they look more like a turnip in color), you can substitute 2 medium/large white daikon radishes (the ones that look more like white carrots). Look for fatter ones that will be easier to cut into noodles.

1. Preheat the oven to 425°F.

2. Use a spiralizer or other noodle-cutting tool to cut the daikon into noodles. You can leave the noodles long or roughly chop them into shorter segments. Place them in a large bowl. Add the onion and use your hands to toss the vegetables together. Pour the avocado oil over the vegetables and toss well. Sprinkle in the hemp hearts, flaxseeds, and ¼ teaspoon of the salt. Toss again until the vegetables are well coated with the seeds.

3. Transfer the mixture to a large, heavy rimmed baking sheet and spread it out as evenly as possible. Scrape out any of the seed mixture stuck to the bowl and sprinkle it over the vegetables. Sprinkle with the remaining ¼ teaspoon salt.

4. Bake until the edges of the vegetables are starting to brown, 25 to 30 minutes. Remove from the oven and toss the mixture with tongs. Transfer to a serving bowl. Scrape up any seed mixture that remains in the pan and sprinkle it over the vegetables.

Mix it up! After mixing all the ingredients in step 2, divide the noodles evenly among 8 silicone muffin cups and gently press them into the bottom. Bake as described. Allow them to cool for a couple minutes, then gently remove them from the muffin cups to serve. Serve with the World's Easiest Dipping Sauce (page 183) or Aioli (page 262).

PESTO VEGGIE FRITTERS

The underappreciated broccoli stem has all sorts of potential once you peel away the woody outer layer: salads, slaws, frittatas, and, of course, fritters. Top these fritters with sour cream or Aioli (page 262) for a little extra fat.

MAKES 12 FRITTERS

1 large zucchini, shredded (about 2 cups)

Kosher salt

1 cup shredded Parmesan cheese

2 tablespoons almond meal (not blanched almond flour, see Note)

¾ teaspoon Italian Seasoning Blend (page 254)

2 large eggs

2 tablespoons pesto, homemade (page 265) or store-bought

4 small broccoli stems, peeled and shredded (about 1 cup), or 1 cup store-bought broccoli slaw

4 tablespoons salted butter

MACRONUTRIENTS PER FRITTER

CALORIES: 99

FAT: 9 G/81 CALORIES

CARBOHYDRATE: 3 G/ 12 CALORIES

PROTEIN: 4 G/16 CALORIES

1. Place the zucchini in a sieve set over a bowl. Sprinkle with a heaping ¼ teaspoon salt and toss to coat. Let the zucchini sit for 10 minutes to draw out excess water.

2. Meanwhile, in a small food processor, combine the Parmesan, almond meal, Italian seasoning, and ¼ teaspoon salt. Pulse the mixture until it resembles coarse sand.

3. In a small bowl, lightly beat the eggs. Mix in the pesto until fully combined. Add the Parmesan mixture to the eggs, along with another ¼ teaspoon salt if needed, and stir well.

4. Use a large spoon or spatula to press as much water as possible out of the zucchini. Place the zucchini in a clean kitchen towel and wring out as much more water as you can. Stir the zucchini and the shredded broccoli into the egg mixture.

5. Heat a large skillet over medium heat and add about one-third of the butter. When the butter starts to foam, give the fritter batter another stir. Working in batches, scoop about 2 tablespoons of batter for each fritter into the hot butter and flatten to about ½ inch thick. Cook the fritters until nicely browned on the first side, about 5 minutes. Carefully flip them and cook another 3 minutes or so on the second side. Remove them to a plate, melt more butter in the pan, and cook the next batch. Repeat if needed with a third batch. Serve hot.

Note: Almond meal is not usually as fine as almond flour. Trader Joe's sells a good almond meal in the baking section. You can also make it yourself by grinding raw almonds in a food processor until they resemble the texture of fine sand.

JÍCAMA FRIES WITH THE WORLD'S EASIEST DIPPING SAUCE

Raw jícama ("hick-a-mah") sticks are delicious dipped in salsa or Guacamole (page 221), but have you ever tried roasting them? They retain more of their crunch than some other roasted vegetables, and they brown beautifully, developing a nice, mild flavor. The jícama root comes in the produce section as a large round bulb, and it takes some effort to first peel it and then chop it into sticks. The increased popularity of jícama means that many markets now offer presliced jícama in the packaged produce snacks section.

SERVES 4

1   pound jícama, peeled

6   tablespoons avocado oil

1   teaspoon Cajun Seasoning (page 253), or seasoning blend of choice

1   teaspoon kosher salt

World's Easiest Dipping Sauce (recipe follows)

MACRONUTRIENTS PER SERVING (WITHOUT DIPPING SAUCE)

CALORIES: 426

FAT: 43 G/385 CALORIES

CARBOHYDRATE: 10 G/ 40 CALORIES

PROTEIN: 1 G/3 CALORIES

1. Preheat the oven to 425°F.

2. Cut the jícama into sticks about ¼ inch thick.

3. Place the jícama sticks in a large bowl and pour the oil over them. Sprinkle on the seasoning and ½ teaspoon of the salt (reduce or omit if using a seasoning blend that contains salt). Toss well.

4. Spread the jícama sticks in a single layer on a heavy rimmed baking sheet. The sticks should not be touching, so use two baking sheets if necessary. Bake for 20 minutes. Remove them from the oven and use a spatula to flip them. Spread them back out and cook for 10 minutes more. They will still be somewhat crispy. Add another 5 to 10 minutes of cooking time if you want them browned more.

5. Remove from the oven and sprinkle with the remaining ½ teaspoon salt if desired. Transfer the jícama to a serving plate and offer the dipping sauce alongside.

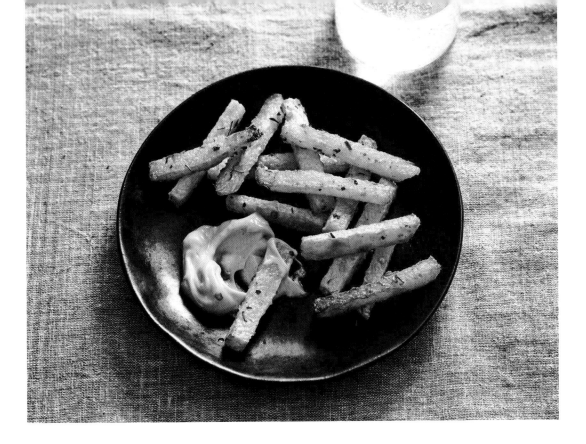

WORLD'S EASIEST DIPPING SAUCE

MAKES ABOUT ⅔ CUP

½   cup Primal Kitchen Chipotle Lime Mayo (see Note)

3   tablespoons full-fat coconut milk

In a small bowl, whisk the mayo and coconut milk together.

Note: To make your own mayo, combine ½ cup avocado oil mayo, 1 additional tablespoon lime juice, ½ teaspoon garlic powder, and ¼ teaspoon chipotle chile powder (or more to taste, but chipotle powder packs a kick). If you can't find chipotle chile powder, use ¾ teaspoon ancho chile powder instead.

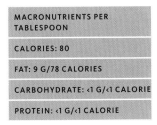

MACRONUTRIENTS PER TABLESPOON

CALORIES: 80

FAT: 9 G/78 CALORIES

CARBOHYDRATE: <1 G/<1 CALORIE

PROTEIN: <1 G/<1 CALORIE

KETO POUTINE

Poutine is a classic French-Canadian dish traditionally made with French fries piled high and smothered with brown gravy and cheese curds. Of course, French fries and brown gravy (thickened with white flour) are both off the keto menu. However, these are a great substitute for days when you can't get "O Canada" out of your head.

SERVES 4

1 pound daikon radish, peeled and ends trimmed

¼ cup avocado oil

Sea salt and ground black pepper

2 tablespoons bacon fat, beef tallow, or fat of choice

1 cup sliced cremini mushrooms (3 ounces)

¼ cup diced onion

½ cup riced cauliflower

1 teaspoon Primal-cestershire Sauce (page 264)

1½ cups beef or chicken bone broth, homemade (page 35) or store-bought

½ teaspoon dried oregano

2 tablespoons unsalted butter

1 cup cheese curds

1. Preheat the oven to 450°F.

2. Cut the daikon into French fry shapes about ¼ inch thick. Place them in a pile on a large, heavy rimmed baking sheet and drizzle them with the avocado oil. Toss with your hands to coat, then spread them out in a single layer so they are not touching. Sprinkle with ¼ teaspoon salt and ⅛ teaspoon pepper. Place them in the hot oven and set a timer for 15 minutes.

3. Meanwhile, start the gravy. In a large pan, heat the bacon fat over medium heat. Add the mushrooms and onion. Cook until they start to brown, about 5 minutes. Add the cauliflower and cook for another 4 minutes. Stir in the primal-cestershire sauce, broth, and oregano. When the liquid comes to a boil, reduce to a gentle simmer, stirring occasionally, while the daikon roasts.

4. When your oven timer beeps, remove the baking sheet from the oven and use a spatula to flip the fries. Sprinkle with additional salt and pepper and return the pan to the oven until the fries are browned, 10 to 15 minutes longer.

5. Remove the fries from the oven. Add the butter to the gravy and stir until melted. Use an immersion blender to blend the mixture until smooth. (Alternatively, carefully transfer the mixture to a regular blender, blend until smooth, and return to the pan.) If the gravy is too thick, stir in a little bit of water or broth. Taste and season with salt and pepper.

6. Position a rack about 6 inches from the broiler. Heat the broiler to low. Crowd the fries into the center of the baking sheet (or transfer them to a broilerproof pan or cast-iron skillet if your baking sheet can't go under the broiler). Ladle about half the gravy evenly over the fries and sprinkle the cheese curds over the top. Broil the fries, watching carefully, until the cheese curds start to brown and melt, about 2 minutes. Remove from the broiler and use a large spatula to transfer the fries to individual serving bowls. Pour any gravy that remains in the pan over the fries, then ladle the remaining reserved gravy over the fries and serve hot.

Note: There are agents you can use to thicken gravy, such as guar gum, tapioca starch, and xantham gum. They are technically keto-approved, but they can also yield an unpleasant texture. Using cauliflower is an easy way to incorporate more veggies in your diet, too.

MACRONUTRIENTS PER SERVING

CALORIES: 327

FAT: 28 G/256 CALORIES

CARBOHYDRATE: 10 G/ 39 CALORIES

PROTEIN: 10 G/38 CALORIES

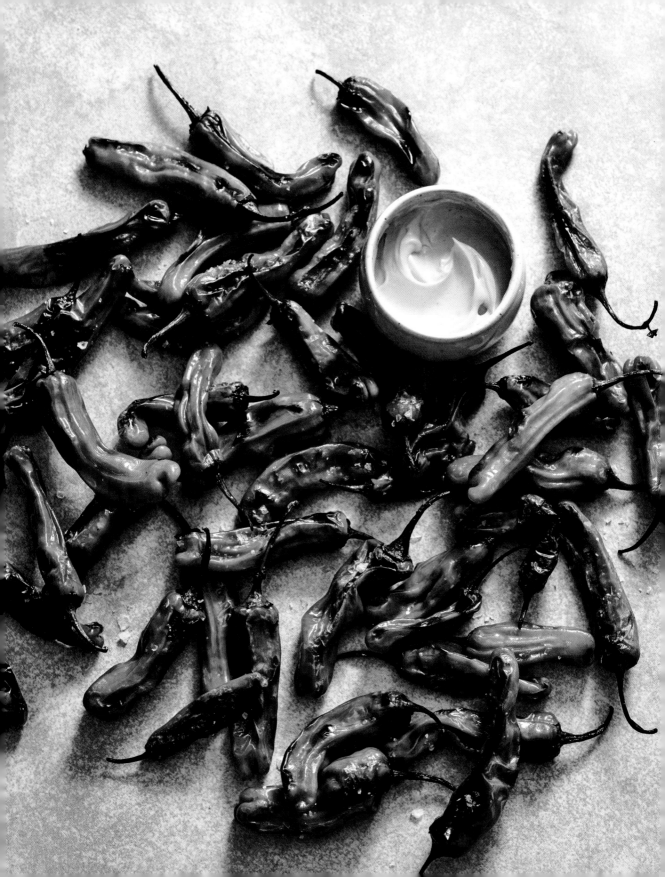

BLISTERED SHISHITO PEPPERS

Shishito peppers are generally pretty mild, but be aware that one out of every ten or so packs a punch. It's like chile pepper roulette—what a fun party game!

SERVES 6

3 tablespoons avocado oil

¾ pound shishito peppers

1 to 1½ teaspoons flaky sea salt

Double recipe of World's Easiest Dipping Sauce (page 183)

MACRONUTRIENTS PER SERVING
CALORIES: 352
FAT: 36 G/328 CALORIES
CARBOHYDRATE: 5 G/ 18 CALORIES
PROTEIN: 1 G/5 CALORIES

In a large cast-iron skillet, heat the avocado oil over medium-high heat. When the oil starts to smoke, add a batch of peppers (only enough to form a single layer in the pan). Cook without disturbing for 2 minutes. Toss and cook another minute. Continue to cook and toss occasionally until the peppers are well browned on all sides, 5 to 7 minutes. Remove to a serving bowl and sprinkle with a generous pinch of flaky salt. Repeat with the rest of the shishito peppers. Serve the dipping sauce in a ramekin alongside the peppers.

TURNIP KOHLRABI GRATIN

This recipe hits the home-cooking, comfort-food spot. It is the perfect side dish for a holiday ham or turkey, and it also makes a great substitute for cheesy breakfast potatoes. Serve this at your next keto brunch and soak in the rave reviews.

SERVES 6

1 tablespoon butter or ghee, melted, or fat of choice

1 heaping cup grated Gruyère cheese

2 cups heavy whipping cream

1 teaspoon kosher salt

½ teaspoon ground black pepper

¼ teaspoon dried thyme

¼ teaspoon dried marjoram or ground nutmeg

1 pound small turnips, peeled and thinly sliced

2 small bulbs kohlrabi, peeled and thinly sliced (see Note)

1 small onion, very thinly sliced

½ cup grated Parmesan cheese

1. Preheat the oven to 400°F. Grease the bottom and sides of an oval gratin dish with the melted butter.

2. Set aside about 2 tablespoons of the Gruyère cheese and add the rest to a large bowl, along with the cream, salt, pepper, thyme, and marjoram. Stir well. Add the turnips, kohlrabi, and onion to the cream mixture. Toss gently to coat the sliced vegetables, trying not to break them.

3. Transfer the mixture to the prepared gratin dish, making sure that the cheese gets more or less evenly distributed throughout. When all the vegetables are in the dish, pour any remaining heavy cream mixture over the top.

4. Mix together the reserved Gruyère cheese and the Parmesan and sprinkle it over the top of the gratin.

5. Bake until the gratin is bubbling and the cheese topping is nicely browned, about 1 hour. Allow the gratin to sit for 10 minutes before serving.

Note: If you can't find kohlrabi, you can substitute daikon radish, rutabaga, or simply add more turnips.

MACRONUTRIENTS PER SERVING

CALORIES: 466

FAT: 41 G/369 CALORIES

CARBOHYDRATE: 11 G/ 44 CALORIES

PROTEIN: 16 G/64 CALORIES

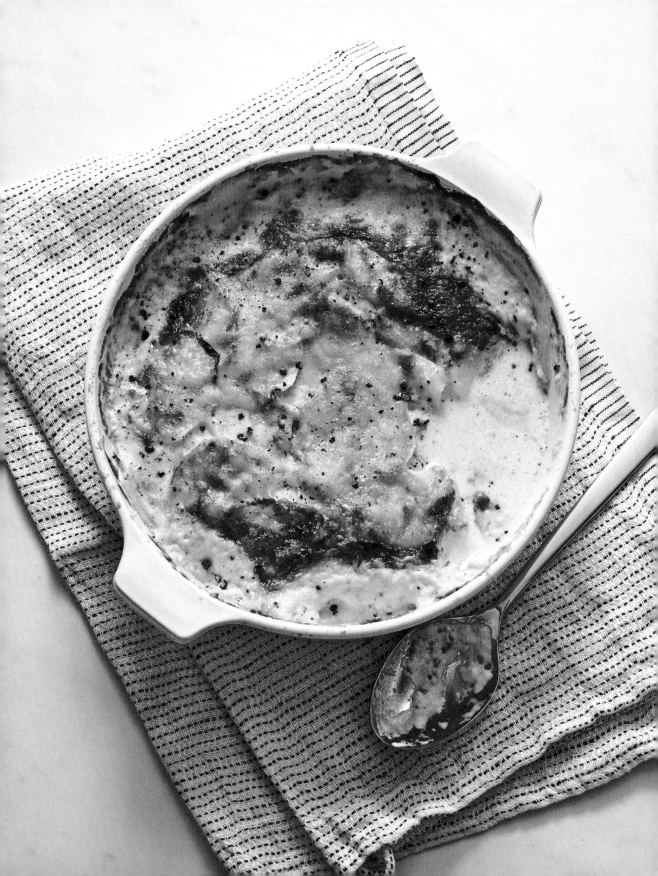

SPAGHETTI SQUASH CARBONARA

Spaghetti squash is a favorite "primal swap." Frankly, it's tastier—and of course much healthier—than regular noodles. With the addition of pancetta, which is similar to bacon, plus egg and cheese, this is quite a hearty side dish. You could even eat it as your main course.

SERVES 4

1 large spaghetti squash

1 tablespoon avocado oil (optional, if baking the squash)

Sea salt and ground black pepper

2 teaspoons bacon fat, or fat of choice

4 ounces pancetta, cubed

1 large egg

¾ cup shredded Parmesan cheese

2 tablespoons chopped fresh parsley

1 tablespoon high-quality extra-virgin olive oil

MACRONUTRIENTS PER SERVING
CALORIES: 307
FAT: 25 G/225 CALORIES
CARBOHYDRATE: 10 G/ 40 CALORIES
PROTEIN: 11 G/44 CALORIES

1. Carefully halve the spaghetti squash through the equator, like a belt (this is easier and safer than attempting to halve the squash lengthwise). Scoop out and discard the seeds. Cook the spaghetti squash according to one of the following methods:

OVEN

a. Preheat the oven to 425°F.

b. Brush the inside of the spaghetti squash with the avocado oil and sprinkle with ½ teaspoon each salt and pepper. Place the spaghetti squash cut side down in a glass baking dish. Bake until a knife easily pierces the skin, about 40 minutes. Remove from the oven and proceed to step 4.

INSTANT POT

a. Pour 1 cup water into the Instant Pot. Place the metal steam rack/trivet or steaming basket inside. Place the spaghetti squash cut side down on the rack or steamer. (If necessary, cut the halves of the spaghetti squash in half again to fit; do not worry if the pieces overlap.) Secure the lid and set the steam release valve to Sealing.

b. Press the Manual button and set the cook time to 7 minutes. When the Instant Pot beeps, carefully switch the steam release valve to Venting to quick-release the pressure. Remove the spaghetti squash from the Instant Pot and proceed to step 4.

2. While the spaghetti squash cooks, heat a skillet over medium heat and melt the bacon fat. Add the pancetta to the hot skillet and cook until crispy, 4 to 5 minutes. Remove the pancetta to a bowl and set aside.

3. Shortly before the spaghetti squash is done, crack the egg into a small bowl and lightly beat it. Stir in ½ teaspoon salt and ¼ teaspoon pepper.

4. When the spaghetti squash is done, carefully use a fork to separate it into strands. Place the strands on a clean kitchen towel. Place a second clean towel on top and gently press down on the spaghetti squash with a cutting board to squeeze some of the excess (hot!) water out of the noodles.

5. Transfer the noodles to a large bowl. Pour the beaten egg over the hot spaghetti squash and toss quickly to coat the noodles before the egg cooks. Add the cooked pancetta, half the Parmesan cheese, and the parsley and toss again. Drizzle with the olive oil and sprinkle with the remaining Parmesan. Serve hot.

KETO COLCANNON

Colcannon is a traditional Irish dish usually made with potatoes and cabbage mashed together with milk and butter. With a few tweaks, it is possible to make a very good version of the dish using only keto-friendly ingredients. You can omit the daikon and add more cauliflower, but the daikon makes the final dish more potatoy.

SERVES 8

- 2 medium daikon radishes, peeled and cut into chunks (about 3 cups)
- 1 large head cauliflower, cut into florets
- 2 leeks, white and light-green parts only
- 6 tablespoons salted butter
- 2 cloves garlic, minced
- 2 cups shredded napa or savoy cabbage (or kale, any variety)
- 1 (13.5-ounce) can full-fat coconut milk or 1½ cups heavy whipping cream
- 2 to 3 teaspoons kosher salt, to taste
- 1 teaspoon ground black pepper

1. Place a steamer basket in a large stockpot and add water to touch the bottom of the steamer basket. Bring the water to a boil. Place the daikon in the steamer, then place the cauliflower on top of the daikon. Cover the pot and steam until the the cauliflower is fork-tender, about 15 minutes.

2. While the cauliflower and daikon steam, quarter the leeks lengthwise. Rinse very well under running water, then thinly slice.

3. In a large skillet, melt 3 tablespoons of the butter over medium heat. Add the leeks and sauté until soft, about 8 minutes. Add the garlic and sauté until the leeks and garlic are browned, another 2 minutes. Stir in the cabbage and coconut milk. Allow the milk to come to a boil, then reduce the heat to a low simmer to thicken the sauce while the cauliflower finishes cooking.

4. When the cauliflower is tender, use a large spoon to remove the florets to a clean kitchen towel. Transfer the daikon radishes to the pan with the cabbage mixture. (It's okay if the cauliflower and daikon get a little mixed up.) Roll up the cauliflower in the kitchen towel. Place a cutting board on top and gently press down to squeeze excess water out of the cauliflower. Add the cauliflower to the rest of the ingredients.

5. Use a potato masher to smash the cauliflower and daikon. (You can also use an immersion blender, but do not

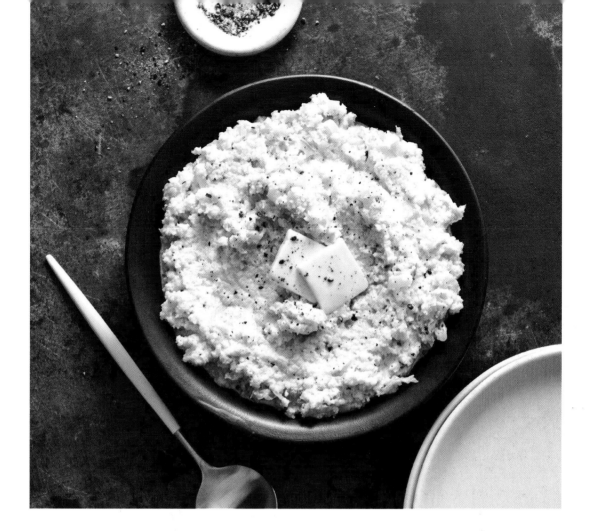

MACRONUTRIENTS PER SERVING

CALORIES: 143

FAT: 10 G/90 CALORIES

CARBOHYDRATE: 13 G/
52 CALORIES

PROTEIN: 3 G/12 CALORIES

overprocess. You want some texture to remain.) Season with the salt and pepper.

6. Transfer the colcannon to a serving bowl. Cut the remaining 3 tablespoons butter into pats and place them on top of the colcannon. Serve hot.

Mix it up! Bacon makes everything better (obviously!), but it is especially great in colcannon. Start by cooking the bacon in the pan you will use for the colcannon. Set the bacon aside, and use the rendered bacon fat to cook the leeks and cabbage instead of the butter in step 3. After mashing the cauliflower and turnips in step 5, crumble the bacon and stir it into the colcannon, reserving a little bit to sprinkle on top before serving.

ZUCCHINI CAULI-FREDO

Alfredo sauce can actually be keto-friendly, but this version is for keto-ers who avoid dairy, or those who simply want to pack more veggies into their diets.

SERVES 4

2   cups cauliflower florets

1   small clove garlic, smashed

¼   cup nutritional yeast

2   tablespoons extra-virgin olive oil

1   tablespoon full-fat coconut milk, nut milk, or water

½   teaspoon fresh lemon juice

½   teaspoon Italian Seasoning Blend (optional; page 254)

1   teaspoon kosher salt

½   teaspoon ground black pepper

2   tablespoons avocado oil

8   ounces cremini mushrooms, sliced

2   small zucchini, halved lengthwise and cut into ½-inch-thick half-moons

¼   cup loosely packed fresh parsley leaves, finely chopped (optional)

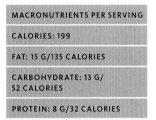

MACRONUTRIENTS PER SERVING
CALORIES: 199
FAT: 15 G/135 CALORIES
CARBOHYDRATE: 13 G/ 52 CALORIES
PROTEIN: 8 G/32 CALORIES

1. In a large pot fitted with a steamer basket, bring 1 to 2 inches of water to a boil. Place the cauliflower and garlic in the steamer basket, cover, and steam until the cauliflower is fork-tender, about 15 minutes.

2. Transfer the cauliflower and garlic to a blender or food processor. Pulse a few times to chop. Add the nutritional yeast, olive oil, coconut milk, lemon juice, Italian seasoning (if using), ½ teaspoon of the salt, and ¼ teaspoon of the pepper. Blend until smooth. Scrape down the sides of the blender and pulse a few more times. Set the cauli-fredo sauce aside.

3. In a large skillet, heat the avocado oil over medium-high heat. When hot, add the mushrooms and sauté until soft, about 4 minutes. Add the zucchini and season with the remaining ½ teaspoon salt and ¼ teaspoon pepper. Cook, stirring frequently, until the zucchini is just soft, about 4 minutes more.

4. Pour the cauli-fredo sauce from the blender over the mushrooms and zucchini. Stir well. Heat until the sauce just starts to bubble, then remove from the heat. Serve garnished with fresh parsley if desired.

Mix it up! If you'd rather make zucchini noodles, make the cauli-fredo as described. Sauté the mushrooms until soft, about 8 minutes. Add the raw zucchini noodles to the mushrooms and sauté for 1 minute. Stir the cauli-fredo sauce into the mushrooms and zucchini, and cook just until the zucchini noodles and sauce are heated through. The zucchini noodles should still be "al dente."

TURNIP NOODLES WITH DANDELION PESTO

Pesto is an easy and delicious way to get both more greens and more healthy fats into a keto diet. Dandelion greens are pleasantly bitter and stand up well against the slightly peppery, slightly sweet flavor of the turnip noodles.

SERVES 4

3 large turnips, peeled and ends trimmed

3 tablespoons avocado oil

Kosher salt and ground black pepper

¼ cup pumpkin seeds or pine nuts

¼ cup walnuts

3 cloves garlic, roughly chopped

¼ cup grated Parmesan cheese

2 cups dandelion greens, stems removed, or arugula

½ cup fresh basil leaves

1 tablespoon fresh lemon juice

⅓ to ½ cup extra-virgin olive oil

MACRONUTRIENTS PER SERVING*

CALORIES: 408

FAT: 39 G/351 CALORIES

CARBOHYDRATE: 12 G/ 48 CALORIES

PROTEIN: 7 G/28 CALORIES

* Macros based on using ⅓ cup olive oil.

1. Preheat the oven to 450°F.

2. Cut the turnip into noodles using a spiralizer or other noodle-cutting tool. Place the noodles on a large, heavy rimmed baking sheet. Drizzle the avocado oil over the noodles and toss to coat. Sprinkle with ½ teaspoon each salt and pepper. Roast until the turnips are al dente, about 10 minutes. If you want them softer, roast another 5 minutes, or until they reach the desired doneness.

3. Meanwhile, in a food processor, combine the pumpkin seeds, walnuts, and garlic and process until the mixture resembles very coarse sand. Add the Parmesan and ¼ teaspoon each salt and pepper. Pulse several times to combine. Add the dandelion greens, basil, and lemon juice. Process until the leaves are chopped very finely.

4. Scrape down the sides with a spatula, then with the food processor running, slowly pour in the olive oil until the pesto reaches the desired consistency. Taste and adjust the salt and pepper.

5. When the turnip noodles are cooked, transfer them to a large bowl. Add the pesto to the noodles and toss very well with tongs until the noodles are coated with pesto. Serve warm or at room temperature.

STOVETOP UN-STUFFING WITH OYSTERS

Obviously this recipe can replace the bread stuffing that traditionally accompanies American Thanksgiving dinners, but
it is meant to be enjoyed year-round. If you are not a fan of
oysters, you can omit them, but they are an excellent source
of many vitamins and minerals, including vitamins D and B$_{12}$,
zinc, and selenium. You can double (or triple!) this recipe to
feed a crowd.

SERVES 4

1 tablespoon avocado oil or fat of choice

1 large daikon radish, peeled and cut into ½-inch cubes

2 medium turnips, peeled and cut into ½-inch cubes

1 medium onion, chopped

2 stalks celery with leaves, cut into ¼-inch slices

2 tablespoons unsalted butter, ghee, or fat of choice

1 pound mushrooms, stems removed and halved if small or quartered if large

1 teaspoon kosher salt

1 teaspoon dried thyme

1 teaspoon dried sage

½ teaspoon ground rosemary

1. In a large skillet, heat the avocado oil over medium heat. Turn the heat down a smidge and add the daikon radish. Cook, stirring frequently, for 5 minutes. Add the turnips, onion, and celery and cook, stirring frequently, until the vegetables are starting to become soft, but are not yet cooked through, about 5 minutes more.

2. Add the butter to the pan and let it melt. Bump the heat back to medium and add the mushrooms. In a small bowl, mix together the salt, thyme, sage, rosemary, marjoram, pepper, and nutmeg. Add the herb/spice mixture to the vegetables in the skillet. Stir well and cook until the mushrooms are soft, about 5 minutes more.

3. Reserving the oil from the cans, drain the oysters and chop into smaller pieces if desired. Add the oysters and the oil to the pan. Add the broth and stir well, scraping the pan to

loosen any browned bits stuck on the bottom. Cook until the oysters are warmed through. Taste the radishes and turnips to make sure they are soft. If not, cook a few more minutes.

4. Transfer the mixture to a serving dish. Stir in the pecans and parsley (if using) immediately before serving. Serve warm.

Note: If you do not have marjoram, you can substitute oregano.

¼ teaspoon dried marjoram (see Note)

¼ teaspoon ground black pepper

⅛ teaspoon ground nutmeg

2 (3-ounce) cans smoked oysters packed in olive oil

¼ cup chicken or turkey bone broth, homemade (page 35) or store-bought

¼ cup pecans, chopped (optional)

3 tablespoons fresh parsley leaves, finely chopped (optional)

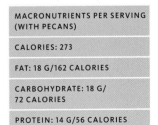

MACRONUTRIENTS PER SERVING (WITH PECANS)

CALORIES: 273

FAT: 18 G/162 CALORIES

CARBOHYDRATE: 18 G/ 72 CALORIES

PROTEIN: 14 G/56 CALORIES

STIR-FRIED BOK CHOY

If bok choy isn't already a staple of your diet, it probably should be. It is one of the most nutrient-dense vegetables you can find, and is thought to have anticancer properties. Among the cruciferous vegetables, it is one of the quickest and easiest to cook, too. Stir-frying is a common cooking method that lets the delicate flavor and texture of bok choy shine.

SERVES 4

FOR THE DRESSING

- ¼ cup fresh cilantro leaves
- 1 clove garlic, smashed
- 1 teaspoon coconut vinegar or apple cider vinegar
- ¼ cup extra-virgin olive oil or avocado oil
- 1 tablespoon sesame oil
- ⅛ teaspoon red pepper flakes (optional)
- Pinch of kosher salt
- Ground black pepper

FOR THE STIR-FRY

- 1 pound baby bok choy, thoroughly washed and ends trimmed
- 1 tablespoon coconut aminos or tamari
- 1 tablespoon coconut vinegar or apple cider vinegar
- 1 tablespoon coconut oil or avocado oil
- 2 cloves garlic, minced
- 1 tablespoon minced fresh ginger

1. For the dressing: In a small food processor, or in a jar that tightly fits your immersion blender, combine the cilantro, garlic, vinegar, olive oil, sesame oil, pepper flakes (if using), salt, and black pepper to taste. Pulse them together until the cilantro is very finely chopped. This can be done a day ahead and refrigerated. Remove it from the refrigerator and allow it to come to room temperature before serving.

2. For the stir-fry: Shake excess water from the bok choy and pat dry. If the bok choy are large, halve them lengthwise through the core.

3. In a small bowl, combine the coconut aminos and vinegar. Set aside.

4. Heat a wok or large, deep skillet with a lid over medium-high heat for 3 to 4 minutes. Add the coconut oil and push it around with a wooden spoon as it melts to coat the bottom of the pan.

5. Add the garlic and ginger and stir-fry until fragrant, about 20 seconds. Add the bok choy (careful, it might splatter) and stir for 2 minutes. Pour the coconut amino mixture over the bok choy and stir-fry for 30 seconds. Cover the pan and let the bok choy steam for another 30 seconds.

6. Transfer the bok choy to a serving plate. Drizzle the dressing over the bok choy. Sprinkle with sesame seeds or crushed nuts if desired. Serve hot.

2   teaspoons toasted sesame seeds, or 2 tablespoons crushed almonds or cashews

MACRONUTRIENTS PER SERVING (WITH SESAME SEEDS)
CALORIES: 177
FAT: 18 G/163 CALORIES
CARBOHYDRATE: 3 G/ 12 CALORIES
PROTEIN: 2 G/10 CALORIES

TAHINI BROCCOLI SALAD

Broccoli salad is great because you can make it ahead of time, and it actually gets better as it sits in the refrigerator. While traditional creamy broccoli salad is delicious, this one might be even better, with a tahini dressing that boasts not only delicious flavor but also the touted anti-inflammatory benefits of turmeric and garlic.

SERVES 4

- 4   cups bite-size broccoli florets
- ¼   cup tahini
- ¼   cup fresh lemon juice
- ¼   cup extra-virgin olive oil
- ½   teaspoon ground cumin
- ¼   teaspoon ground turmeric
- ¼   teaspoon ground black pepper
        Kosher salt
- 1   large clove garlic, pressed or very finely minced
- 1   small shallot, very finely minced
- ¼   cup chopped salted pistachios or slivered almonds

MACRONUTRIENTS PER SERVING

CALORIES: 294

FAT: 26 G/230 CALORIES

CARBOHYDRATE: 14 G/ 56 CALORIES

PROTEIN: 7 G/28 CALORIES

1. In a large pot fitted with a steamer basket, bring 1 to 2 inches of water to a boil. Fill a large bowl with ice water. Place the broccoli in the steamer basket, cover, and steam for 2 minutes, just until the broccoli turns bright green. You want it to retain some crunchiness. Transfer the broccoli to the ice bath. Let it sit for a minute to stop the cooking.

2. Drain the broccoli in a strainer or colander. Shake off as much excess water as possible. Pat the broccoli dry with a clean kitchen towel.

3. In a large bowl, combine the tahini, lemon juice, olive oil, cumin, turmeric, pepper, ½ teaspoon salt, the garlic, and shallot. Taste and adjust the salt.

4. Add the broccoli to the dressing and stir very well to coat the broccoli. Refrigerate for 1 hour to chill. You can also make this salad a day ahead.

5. Before serving, let the salad sit at room temperature for a few minutes, then stir it well. Sprinkle it with the pistachios and serve cool or at room temperature.

BUTTER-BRAISED RADISHES

If you have only ever had raw radishes, you're in for a treat with this recipe. Cooked radishes are surprisingly delicate in flavor compared to their raw counterparts. You might even confuse them for potatoes if you didn't know better.

SERVES 4

3 bunches radishes with leaves

3 tablespoons unsalted butter

1 tablespoon extra-virgin olive oil

½ teaspoon kosher salt

¼ teaspoon ground black pepper

½ cup chicken bone broth, homemade (page 35) or store-bought, or vegetable stock

MACRONUTRIENTS PER SERVING
CALORIES: 135
FAT: 13 G/113 CALORIES
CARBOHYDRATE: 5 G/ 20 CALORIES
PROTEIN: 2 G/7 CALORIES

1. Trim the ends off the radishes. If they are small, cut them in half. If they are larger, cut them into 3 or 4 pieces. Save the radish tops.

2. In a large skillet, heat 2 tablespoons of butter and the olive oil. When the butter starts to foam, add the radishes in as close to a single layer as possible. Season with the salt and pepper. Cover and cook for 4 minutes. Uncover, stir the radishes, and pour in the broth. Bring the liquid to a boil, then reduce to a simmer, cover, and cook until radishes are tender, another 6 to 8 minutes.

3. Meanwhile, wash the radish tops very well. Cut off about 2 tablespoons of leaves, pat them dry with a clean kitchen towel, and finely chop them.

4. Use a slotted spoon to remove the radishes to a serving bowl. Increase the heat to medium-high and whisk the remaining 1 tablespoon butter and the chopped radish leaves into the cooking liquid. Cook, whisking constantly, to slightly thicken the sauce, about 2 minutes. Pour the liquid over the radishes and serve hot.

APPETIZERS & SMALL BITES

BROCCOLI BITES, CRACKERS, AND BUNS

What is there to say about a broccoli and cheese dish that can also be used as *bread* for your favorite sandwiches or sliders? Nothing except: TRY THIS!

MAKES 12 BITES OR CRACKERS, OR 4 BUNS

2 cups broccoli florets

½ cup shredded mozzarella cheese

½ cup shredded Parmesan cheese

¾ teaspoon kosher salt

½ teaspoon ground black pepper

¼ teaspoon garlic powder

MACRONUTRIENTS PER SERVING
(3 BITES OR 1 BUN)

CALORIES: 114

FAT: 7 G/63 CALORIES

CARBOHYDRATE: 5 G/
20 CALORIES

PROTEIN: 8 G/32 CALORIES

1. Preheat the oven to 400°F. Line a large rimmed baking sheet with parchment paper.

2. In a large pot fitted with a steamer basket, bring 1 to 2 inches of water to a boil. Fill a large bowl with ice water. Place the broccoli in the steamer, cover, and steam for 3 minutes. Transfer the broccoli immediately to the ice bath. Let it sit for a minute to stop the cooking, then drain very well in a sieve or colander. Place the broccoli on a clean kitchen towel and pat dry.

3. In a food processor, combine the broccoli, mozzarella, Parmesan, salt, pepper, and garlic powder. Pulse about 10 times to chop, but do not grind it too finely.

4. For bites or crackers, scoop heaping tablespoons of the mixture onto the prepared baking sheet and press down slightly to form "cookies." For buns, scoop 3 tablespoons of the broccoli mixture into your hand and gently squeeze into a ball; place it on the prepared baking sheet and gently flatten. (In either case, the bites or buns will flatten more as they bake.) Bake until browned around the edges and on top, for 22 to 25 minutes. Remove the baking sheet from the oven and let sit for 5 minutes before removing the bites or buns from the baking sheet with a spatula. Serve warm or at room temperature.

BACON PARTY MIX

Try not to eat the whole bowl in one sitting—remember it's called a party mix!

SERVES 12

4	slices sugar-free bacon
1	egg white
1	tablespoon water
1	cup almonds
1	cup cashews
½	cup walnuts
½	cup hazelnuts
¾	teaspoon sweet paprika
¾	teaspoon ground coriander
¾	teaspoon ground cumin
¾	teaspoon ground turmeric
½	teaspoon sea salt
	Cayenne pepper (optional)
½	cup unsweetened coconut flakes
¼	teaspoon ground cinnamon

MACRONUTRIENTS PER SERVING

CALORIES: 223

FAT: 19 G/175 CALORIES

CARBOHYDRATE: 8 G/ 33 CALORIES

PROTEIN: 7 G/29 CALORIES

1. Preheat the oven to 400°F.

2. Place the bacon on a large rimmed baking sheet so the slices are not touching. Bake until crispy, 20 to 25 minutes. Use tongs to remove the bacon to a plate to cool. Reserve the bacon fat for step 5.

3. Reduce the oven temperature to 300°F.

4. In a large bowl, whisk the egg white and water until frothy. Add the nuts and mix well to coat. Place the nuts in a sieve and place the sieve over a second bowl or in the sink. Allow the nuts to drain for 2 to 3 minutes, stirring a couple times. Discard the egg white that drains off.

5. Return the nuts to the large bowl. Add the paprika, coriander, cumin, turmeric, salt, and ¼ teaspoon cayenne (if using). Pour in the reserved bacon fat from the baking sheet and mix well again.

6. Spread the nuts in a single layer on the same baking sheet the bacon was cooked on. Roast for 15 minutes. Remove the pan from the oven and use a spatula to toss the nuts. Spread the nuts back out in a single layer and return the pan to the oven to cook until browned and fragrant, another 15 minutes.

7. Meanwhile, in a dry skillet, gently toast the coconut over medium-low heat until lightly brown, being careful not to burn it, about 2 minutes. Transfer the coconut flakes to a large clean bowl and toss with the cinnamon and a pinch of cayenne (if using).

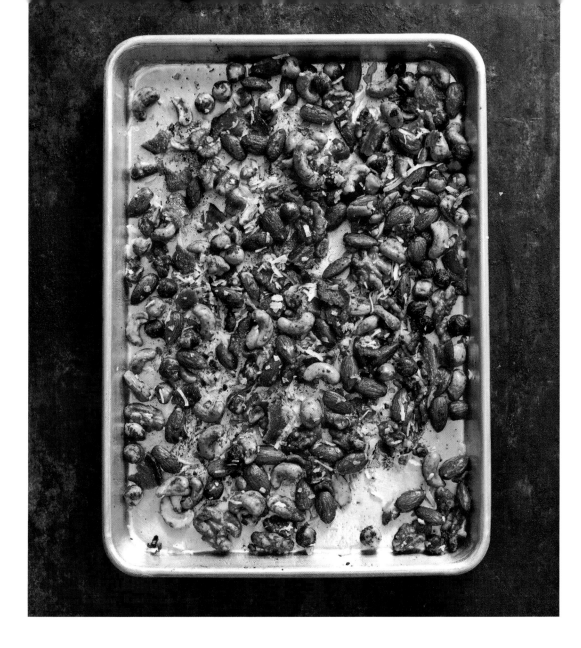

Mix it up! Chop half a bar (about 1.75 ounces/50 g) of very dark chocolate into small pieces. Combine with the trail mix when it is completely cool, or when it is still warm if you want the chocolate to melt slightly over the nuts and bacon.

8. Remove the nuts from the oven and transfer them to the bowl with the coconut. Crumble the bacon into the same bowl and stir everything together. Allow the mixture to cool for 30 minutes, stirring occasionally. Serve immediately, or wait until the nuts are completely cool, then store in an airtight container in the refrigerator.

ROAST BEEF BITES WITH HORSERADISH SAUCE

These bites capture all the flavors of your favorite roast beef dinner, but they take only a few minutes to make. You can use roast beef from the deli, or make these bites with leftovers from your next holiday prime rib.

MAKES 16 SKEWERS

FOR THE DIPPING SAUCE

- ¼ cup heavy whipping cream
- 2 tablespoons full-fat sour cream
- 2 tablespoons avocado oil mayonnaise
- 3 tablespoons prepared horseradish
- 2 teaspoons fresh lemon juice
- 2 teaspoons Dijon mustard, preferably whole-grain
- ¼ teaspoon sea salt
- ¼ teaspoon ground black pepper

FOR THE BITES

- 16 thin slices roast beef
- 32 dill pickle slices

1. Prepare the dipping sauce: Beat the cream until starting to become thick but not yet forming stiff peaks. The easiest way to do this is to use a jar that tightly fits your immersion blender. Blend the whipping cream on low speed for 30 to 45 seconds.

2. In a small bowl, stir together the sour cream, mayo, horseradish, lemon juice, mustard, salt, and pepper. Stir in the whipped cream. Refrigerate until ready to use. This can be done a day ahead.

3. For the bites: Cut the roast beef slices in half. Assemble the bites by folding each piece of roast beef until it is about the same size as the dill pickle slices. On a toothpick skewer, thread a pickle, roast beef, pickle, roast beef. Arrange the skewers on a serving plate and serve with the dipping sauce on the side.

MACRONUTRIENTS PER 4 SKEWERS
CALORIES: 160
FAT: 13 G/120 CALORIES
CARBOHYDRATE: 5 G/ 18 CALORIES
PROTEIN: 7 G/29 CALORIES

EVERYTHING CHEESE BALLS

A great option for a keto party platter or a savory snack. You won't even miss the bagel.

MAKES ABOUT
20 BALLS

- 4 ounces full-fat cream cheese, at room temperature
- ¼ cup full-fat sour cream
- ½ cup shredded Swiss or mozzarella cheese
- 1 teaspoon prepared horseradish
- 1 teaspoon garlic powder
- 1 teaspoon onion powder
- Sea salt
- ¼ teaspoon ground black pepper
- ½ cup toasted sesame seeds (white, black, or a mix)

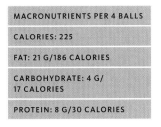

MACRONUTRIENTS PER 4 BALLS

CALORIES: 225

FAT: 21 G/186 CALORIES

CARBOHYDRATE: 4 G/
17 CALORIES

PROTEIN: 8 G/30 CALORIES

1. In a stand mixer (you can also use a hand mixer and bowl), combine the cream cheese, sour cream, Swiss cheese, horseradish, garlic powder, onion powder, ¼ teaspoon salt, and the pepper. Mix on low about 1 minute, until the ingredients are thoroughly combined. Taste and add more salt if needed. Place the mixture in the refrigerator for 10 to 15 minutes to chill.

2. Place the sesame seeds in a small bowl. Scoop out a spoonful of the cheese mixture and roll into a ball using your hands. The ball should be about the size of a large marble. Dip the ball in the sesame seeds and roll to coat. Place the ball on a plate. Repeat with the remaining cheese mixture. Return to the refrigerator to chill until ready to serve.

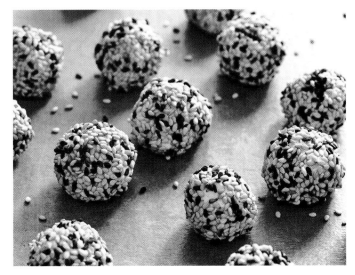

BLUE CHEESE BACON BALLS

The title says everything you need to know here. Bring these to a party if you want to be the most popular one there. Just sayin'.

MAKES ABOUT 24 BALLS

¼ cup almonds

2 tablespoons ground hemp seeds

4 slices sugar-free bacon

4 ounces full-fat cream cheese, at room temperature

½ cup crumbled blue cheese

½ cup shredded white cheddar cheese

2 teaspoons Dijon mustard

¼ teaspoon ground black pepper

MACRONUTRIENTS PER 4 BALLS

CALORIES: 139

FAT: 12 G/112 CALORIES

CARBOHYDRATE: 3 G/ 11 CALORIES

PROTEIN: 5 G/20 CALORIES

1. In a small food processor, pulse the almonds until they are the consistency of coarse sand. Transfer the ground almonds to a cold skillet and add the hemp seeds. Set the skillet over medium heat and toast, stirring frequently, until fragrant and slightly browned, about 4 minutes. Place the mixture in a small bowl and set aside.

2. Use kitchen shears to cut the bacon into small pieces. Cook the bacon in the skillet over medium heat until very crispy, 3 to 5 minutes.

3. Use a spatula to scrape the bacon and the rendered bacon fat into the bowl of a stand mixer (you can also use a hand mixer and bowl). Add the three types of cheese, the mustard, and pepper to the bowl. Mix on low speed until everything is thoroughly combined, about 1 minute. Refrigerate the mixture for 10 to 15 minutes to chill.

4. Scoop out 1 tablespoon at a time of the cheese mixture and roll it into a ball using your hands. Dip the ball in the almond and hemp seed mixture. Roll to coat. Place the ball on a plate. Repeat for the remaining cheese mixture. Return to the refrigerator to chill until ready to serve.

PARMESAN CRISPS

Try this cracker replacement for serving with any dip or pâté, with salami, or just on its own to satisfy a craving for a salty, crunchy snack.

MAKES ABOUT 28 CRISPS

2 cups grated Parmesan cheese

MACRONUTRIENTS PER 7 CRISPS

CALORIES: 210

FAT: 14 G/126 CALORIES

CARBOHYDRATE: 7 G/ 28 CALORIES

PROTEIN: 14 G/56 CALORIES

1. Preheat the oven to 400°F. Line a baking sheet with a silicone mat or parchment paper.

2. Scoop a generous tablespoon of the cheese onto the sheet and flatten it slightly. Repeat with the rest of the cheese, leaving about 1 inch of space in between them. Bake until crisp, 3 to 5 minutes. Allow them to cool completely before serving.

CHOPPED LIVER

Chopped liver is essentially a cross between liver pâté and egg salad. There are countless ways to vary the basic recipe by using different spices, by adding avocado oil mayonnaise for a creamy version, or by mixing in different fats instead of the olive oil. Serve with celery sticks, sliced cucumber, mini sweet peppers (halved), or Parmesan Crisps (page 209).

SERVES 8

2	tablespoons bacon fat or fat of choice
1	onion, finely chopped
1	pound chicken livers, rinsed and patted dry
4	hard-boiled eggs, chopped
1	tablespoon Dijon mustard
2 to 4	tablespoons extra-virgin olive oil
1	teaspoon fine sea salt
½	teaspoon ground black pepper
	Flaky sea salt, for garnish

MACRONUTRIENTS PER SERVING*

CALORIES: 225

FAT: 16 G/145 CALORIES

CARBOHYDRATE: 2 G/9 CALORIES

PROTEIN: 17 G/68 CALORIES

* Macros based on using 4 tablespoons olive oil.

1. In a medium skillet, heat the bacon fat over medium heat. Add the onion and sauté until just soft, about 3 minutes.

2. Add the livers and cook, flipping occasionally, until they are cooked through but still slightly pink in the center, about 7 minutes. Remove the pan from the heat and let the onion and livers cool.

3. Chop the livers into small pieces with a knife and place them in a medium bowl. Add the chopped eggs and stir with a fork. Add the mustard, 2 tablespoons of the olive oil, the fine sea salt, and pepper. Stir well, mashing with the fork. If the texture seems dry, add the rest of the olive oil. Some people prefer the end result to have some texture, others like it totally smooth; continue mashing with the fork until it reaches the desired consistency. Transfer to a large ramekin and sprinkle with flaky salt to serve.

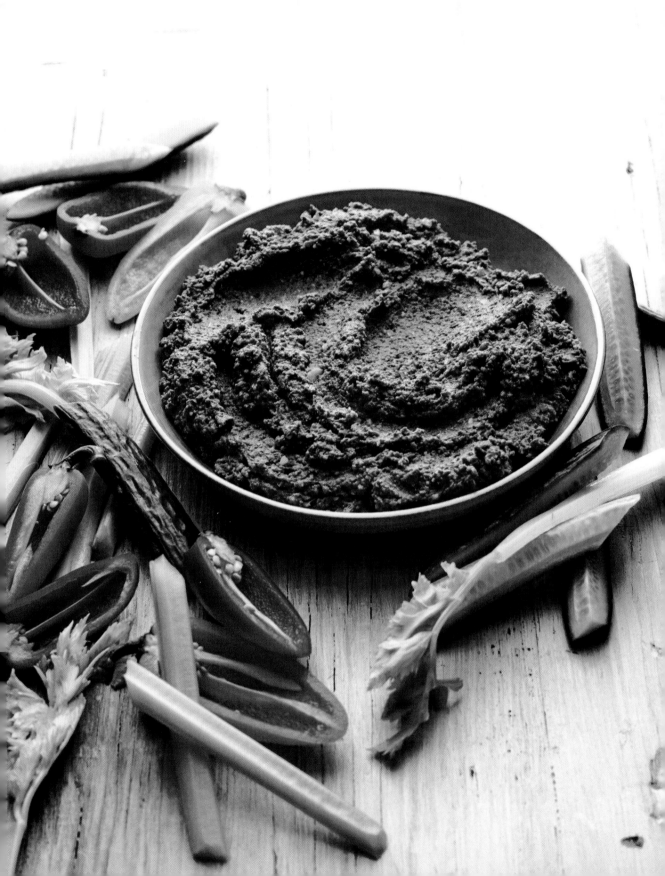

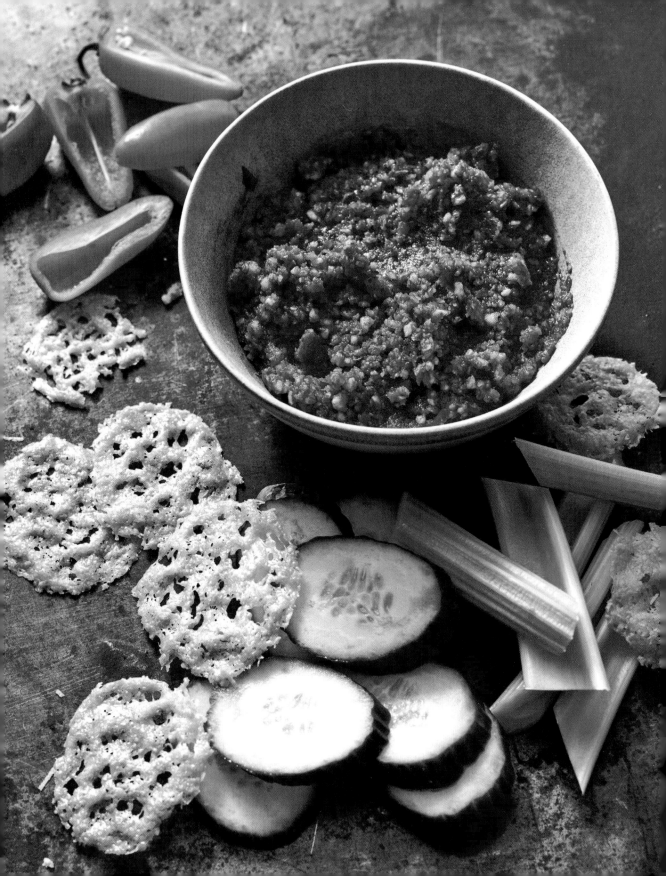

HARISSA ALMOND DIP

Harissa is the generic name for a paste made with chile peppers and olive oil that is a staple of North African cuisines. For this recipe, look for a mild harissa made from red bell peppers instead of hot chiles; but if you are a fan of spicy foods, feel free to experiment with different types of harissa. Serve with sliced vegetables or Parmesan Crisps (page 209), or use it as a spread on lettuce-wrapped meat and cheese "sandwiches."

SERVES 8

¾ cup raw or blanched almonds

¼ cup mild red pepper harissa

Juice of ½ lemon

½ to 1 teaspoon kosher salt

¼ cup good-quality extra-virgin olive oil

MACRONUTRIENTS PER SERVING

CALORIES: 125

FAT: 12 G/108 CALORIES

CARBOHYDRATE: 3 G/ 12 CALORIES

PROTEIN: 2 G/8 CALORIES

1. Preheat the oven to 400°F.

2. Spread the almonds in a single layer on a large rimmed baking sheet. Toast in the oven until they turn darker brown and fragrant (but not burned), 20 to 30 minutes, stirring after 10 minutes. When you can smell them, start watching them carefully!

3. Remove the almonds from the oven and allow them to cool. When they are cool, transfer the almonds to a food processor. Add the harissa, lemon juice, and ½ teaspoon salt. Process until the nuts are ground but the mixture still retains a bit of texture. Taste the mixture and add the remaining salt if needed.

4. With the food processor running, stream in the olive oil and process until the mixture becomes a thick paste, leaving it a little bit chunky. (Or you can continue processing until it is smoother.) Transfer the dip to a serving bowl and serve at room temperature.

CHIPOTLE LIME CAULIFLOWER HUMMUS

Thank you to Jessi Heggan, of Jessi's Kitchen, for this recipe (featured in *The Primal Kitchen Cookbook*)!

SERVES 6

- 1 head cauliflower, cut into florets
- 3 tablespoons avocado oil, plus more for drizzling
- ½ teaspoon smoked paprika, plus more for garnish
- 1¼ teaspoons sea salt
- ⅓ cup Primal Kitchen Chipotle Lime Mayo (see Note, page 183)
- ½ cup fresh cilantro leaves
- 2 tablespoons fresh lime juice
- 1 teaspoon garlic powder

1. Preheat the oven to 400° F. Line a rimmed baking sheet with parchment paper.

2. Place the cauliflower on the baking sheet and toss with avocado oil, paprika, and 1 teaspoon of the salt. Roast the cauliflower until softened and slightly browned, 20 to 25 minutes.

3. In a food processor, combine the roasted cauliflower, mayo, cilantro, lime juice, garlic powder, and remaining ¼ teaspoon salt and blend until the mixture is smooth.

4. Serve immediately while warm, or place in an airtight container to chill in the refrigerator. If desired, drizzle more avocado oil and paprika on top before serving, and enjoy!

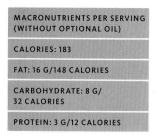

MACRONUTRIENTS PER SERVING (WITHOUT OPTIONAL OIL)

CALORIES: 183

FAT: 16 G/148 CALORIES

CARBOHYDRATE: 8 G/ 32 CALORIES

PROTEIN: 3 G/12 CALORIES

NO-NUT NUTTY BITES

Here's an option for nut-free keto-ers. When shopping for sunflower seed butter, make sure you check the label and select one that is only sunflower seeds (and salt), no sugar added.

2 tablespoons full-fat coconut milk

1 tablespoon chia seeds

4 tablespoons coconut oil, melted

½ cup sunflower seed butter

½ teaspoon ground cinnamon

Pinch of sea salt (if sunflower seed butter is unsalted)

3 to 5 drops liquid stevia, to taste (optional)

3 tablespoons hemp hearts

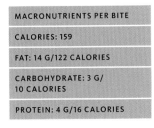

MACRONUTRIENTS PER BITE

CALORIES: 159

FAT: 14 G/122 CALORIES

CARBOHYDRATE: 3 G/ 10 CALORIES

PROTEIN: 4 G/16 CALORIES

1. In a small bowl, mix together the coconut milk and chia seeds and allow the mixture to sit for 10 minutes.

2. Meanwhile, in a separate bowl, combine the coconut oil, sunflower seed butter, ¼ teaspoon cinnamon, the salt, and stevia (if using).

3. Pour the coconut milk and chia seeds into the sunflower seed butter mixture, and stir thoroughly.

4. Heat a small skillet over medium heat. Add the hemp hearts and toast 3 to 4 minutes, stirring frequently and being careful not to let them burn. Transfer the hemp hearts to a small bowl and stir in the remaining ¼ teaspoon cinnamon.

5. Line a plate with wax paper or parchment paper. Use wet hands to roll about 1 heaping tablespoon of the dough into a ball. (If the mixture is too sticky, place it in the freezer for 5 to 10 minutes.) Drop the ball into the hemp hearts and toss to coat. Place the ball on the prepared plate. Repeat for the rest of the dough.

6. Place the balls in the freezer for 30 minutes to harden. Transfer to an airtight container and store in the freezer. Serve straight from the freezer, allowing a couple minutes to sit at room temperature if frozen solid.

GINGER BITES

These evoke your favorite gingerbread cookies but with only simple, keto-friendly ingredients. They are best straight out of the freezer.

MAKES 8 BITES

½ cup raw or toasted pecans

1 tablespoon chia seeds

1 teaspoon pumpkin pie spice, homemade (page 255) or store-bought

1 teaspoon ground ginger

¼ teaspoon sea salt

2 teaspoons erythritol or Lakanto Classic sweetener, or a pinch of stevia powder

¼ cup almond butter (smooth or chunky)

2 tablespoons coconut oil, melted

1. In a food processor, pulse the pecans, chia seeds, pumpkin pie spice, ginger, salt, and the sweetener until the mixture resembles coarse sand. Add the almond butter and coconut oil. Blend for about 10 seconds, until thoroughly combined.

2. Line a small plate with wax paper or parchment paper. Scoop out about 1 heaping teaspoon at a time of the mixture. Use your hands to roll it into a ball and place it on the plate. Repeat for the rest of the mixture. Refrigerate the balls for 30 minutes to harden. Store in an airtight container in the refrigerator or freezer.

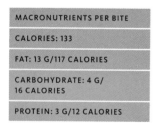

MACRONUTRIENTS PER BITE

CALORIES: 133

FAT: 13 G/117 CALORIES

CARBOHYDRATE: 4 G/ 16 CALORIES

PROTEIN: 3 G/12 CALORIES

KOMBUCHA GUMMIES

If you brew kombucha at home, chances are that you sometimes find yourself with more kombucha than you can drink. If you don't home-brew, you can find kombucha in a variety of flavors at almost any grocery store now. For fun, you can buy silicone molds in the shape of gummy bears or a variety of other shapes, or you can simply use a glass dish and cut the final product into bite-size squares. Adults and kids both enjoy these!

SERVES 6

1 tablespoon coconut oil, melted

¾ cup kombucha (home-brewed or store-bought), any flavor, room temperature

1 to 2 tablespoons grass-fed gelatin powder (see Note)

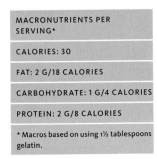

MACRONUTRIENTS PER SERVING*

CALORIES: 30

FAT: 2 G/18 CALORIES

CARBOHYDRATE: 1 G/4 CALORIES

PROTEIN: 2 G/8 CALORIES

* Macros based on using 1½ tablespoons gelatin.

1. Grease a silicone mold in the shape of your choice with the coconut oil. A 6 × 6-inch glass baking dish will also work. If you are using a silicone mold, place it on a small baking sheet.

2. Place the kombucha in a small saucepan and set over *low* heat (you do not want to overheat the kombucha). One teaspoonful at a time, sprinkle the gelatin powder over the surface of the kombucha and whisk it in. When all the gelatin has been incorporated, continue to cook another minute, whisking, until the mixture is smooth. Remove it from the heat and immediately pour the liquid into your prepared pan or mold.

3. Transfer the pan or mold to the refrigerator and chill until the mixture is set, about 2 hours. Remove the gummies from the mold (or if in the baking dish, cut into individual squares) and store them between layers of wax paper or parchment paper in an airtight container in the refrigerator. They will keep for at least 1 week.

Note: 1 tablespoon gelatin is enough to set up the kombucha if using a glass dish or larger silicone molds (e.g., muffin tins), but you might need to increase the gelatin to 1½ to 2 tablespoons if using small silicone molds (e.g., gummy bears). The latter makes them easier to unmold but also denser and chewier. Experiment to find the amount that you prefer.

LEMON PROTEIN BALLS

For staying on track, it can be helpful to keep something like these lemon protein balls on hand to knock down small cravings, or as a keto-friendly snack or exercise fuel. They will soften if not kept cold, so don't make the mistake of sticking them in the pocket of your bike jersey during your next summertime ride. Not that one of us actually did that. . . .

MAKES 12 BALLS

¼ cup coconut oil

2 tablespoons coconut butter

1 cup macadamia nuts

2 tablespoons fresh lemon juice

¼ teaspoon sea salt

2 scoops vanilla-flavored whey protein powder

⅓ cup unsweetened shredded coconut

MACRONUTRIENTS PER BALL*

CALORIES: 182

FAT: 17 G/153 CALORIES

CARBOHYDRATE: 4 G/ 16 CALORIES

PROTEIN: 5 G/20 CALORIES

* Macros based on using Primal Fuel Vanilla Coconut Protein Powder.

1. Place the coconut oil and coconut butter in a microwave-safe bowl. Microwave on high for 25 seconds. Stir and set aside.

2. In a small food processor, process the macadamias for 30 seconds. Scrape down the sides of the bowl and add the melted coconut oil mixture, lemon juice, and salt. Process until the mixture is very smooth. Add the protein powder and pulse about 5 times, until just combined.

3. Use a spatula to scrape the macadamia mixture into a small bowl. Refrigerate the mixture for about 15 minutes to make it easier to handle.

4. Line a plate with wax paper or parchment paper and place the coconut in a small bowl. Scoop out about 1 heaping tea-spoon at a time of the macadamia mixture. Use your hands to roll it into a ball. Drop it in the coconut and roll to coat. Place it on the plate. Repeat for the rest of the macadamia mixture. Place the balls in the freezer for 30 minutes to harden. Store in an airtight container in the freezer. Serve straight from the freezer, allowing a couple minutes for them to sit at room temperature if frozen solid.

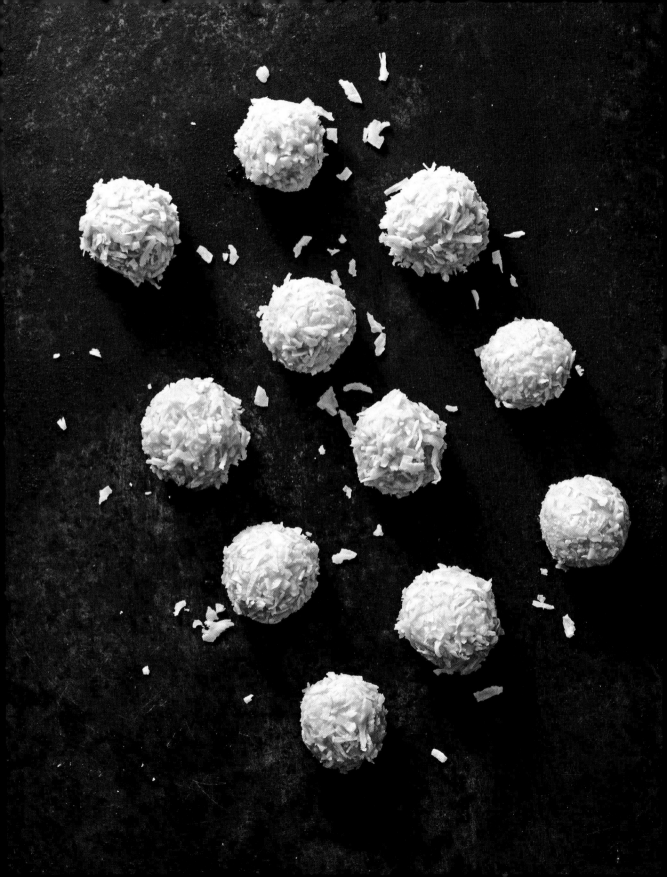

HEAVEN BUTTER

When you taste this, you will understand the name. You will probably end up eating this with a spoon, it's just that good. However, you can also spread this on celery sticks, or put a big dollop inside half an avocado, sprinkle with salt, and eat it before a tough workout. Trust us on this one.

MAKES ABOUT 2 CUPS

1 cup pecans

1 cup hazelnuts

¼ cup unsweetened coconut flakes

2 tablespoons coconut oil, at room temperature

2 tablespoons coconut butter, at room temperature

¼ teaspoon vanilla extract

¼ teaspoon sea salt

2 tablespoons cacao nibs

MACRONUTRIENTS PER 2 TABLESPOONS

CALORIES: 140

FAT: 14 G/128 CALORIES

CARBOHYDRATE: 3 G/ 14 CALORIES

PROTEIN: 2 G/9 CALORIES

1. Preheat the oven to 350°F.

2. Spread the pecans and hazelnuts in a single layer on separate rimmed baking sheets (in case they brown at different rates). Place the nuts in the oven, but do not walk away! Bake until the nuts begin to brown, about 5 minutes. Remove the pecans as soon as you start to smell them. The hazelnuts might need a couple extra minutes. Allow the nuts to cool for 5 to 10 minutes.

3. In a high-powered blender or food processor, blend the nuts on high for 30 seconds. Stop and scrape down the sides, then blend for 30 seconds more. Continue until the nuts are ground into a mostly smooth nut butter (it is okay if some small chunks remain).

4. Add the coconut flakes, coconut oil, coconut butter, vanilla, sea salt, and cacao nibs and blend for 10 seconds. Scrape down the sides again. If you want smoother nut butter, pulse the mixture until it reaches the desired consistency. Place the finished nut butter in an airtight jar and store in the refrigerator. It will keep for several weeks.

GUACAMOLE

A classic. Just hold the chips and try jícama sticks instead! | **SERVES 6**

3 avocados

⅓ cup fresh lime or lemon juice

½ onion, minced

1 tablespoon finely minced serrano chiles (seeds and ribs removed)

1 tablespoon chopped fresh cilantro leaves

Kosher salt

1 medium tomato, seeded and chopped

Scoop the avocado flesh into a medium bowl and mash with a fork. Mix in the lime juice, onion, chiles, cilantro, and 1 teaspoon salt. Gently stir in the tomatoes. Taste and add more salt if desired. Serve immediately.

MACRONUTRIENTS PER SERVING
CALORIES: 125
FAT: 11 G/99 CALORIES
CARBOHYDRATE: 9 G/ 36 CALORIES
PROTEIN: 2 G/8 CALORIES

BAKING & DESSERTS

BASIC BISCUITS

Biscuits—even keto-friendly biscuits—should be considered an "occasional" food in a well-formulated ketogenic diet. Nevertheless, it is nice to have a recipe like this in one's back pocket, especially if you happen to have a delicious sausage gravy recipe . . . (see page 50).

MAKES 6 BISCUITS

4   tablespoons coconut oil, melted

4   large eggs

½   cup full-fat coconut milk

½   teaspoon sea salt

1   tablespoon tapioca starch or arrowroot powder

¼   cup coconut flour

MACRONUTRIENTS PER BISCUIT
CALORIES: 192
FAT: 17 G/153 CALORIES
CARBOHYDRATE: 5 G/ 18 CALORIES
PROTEIN: 5 G/20 CALORIES

1. Preheat the oven to 350°F. Grease 6 cups of a standard muffin tin with 2 tablespoons of the coconut oil, making sure to get the sides of each cup.

2. Crack the eggs into a blender and add the coconut milk and salt. Blend for 10 to 15 seconds to lightly beat.

3. Remove the lid of the blender and place a fine-mesh sieve over the blender jar. Put the tapioca starch and coconut flour in the sieve and stir with a spoon to sift the dry ingredients into the blender. Replace the lid and pulse a few times.

4. Use a spatula to scrape down the sides of the blender. Pour in the remaining 2 tablespoons coconut oil and pulse a few more times to combine.

5. Divide the batter among the 6 greased muffin cups. Bake until the tops appear dry and a toothpick inserted in the center comes out clean, about 25 minutes. Let the biscuits cool in the pan for a few minutes, then run a knife around the edges and use a small spatula to remove them from the tin. Serve warm or at room temperature. Store any leftovers in an airtight container in the refrigerator.

NUT PULP ROLLS
OR HAMBURGER BUNS

One of the things that is cool about making your own nut milk (see page 38) is that you can use the nut pulp left over so that nothing goes to waste. For keto baking, psyllium husk makes a huge difference in the texture of the final product. Look for it in the bulk foods section of your supermarket or in the vitamins and supplements section of a natural foods store.

MAKES 12 ROLLS OR 4 TO 6 BUNS

¼   cup ground psyllium husks

1½ teaspoons baking powder, homemade (page 253) or store-bought

½   teaspoon kosher salt

2   large eggs

½   teaspoon apple cider vinegar

1   tablespoon filtered water

1   tablespoon extra-virgin olive oil

1   cup nut pulp leftover from making nut milk (see page 38)

1   tablespoon toasted sesame seeds (optional)

1. Preheat the oven to 350°F. Line a baking sheet with parchment paper.

2. In a small bowl, stir together the psyllium husks, baking powder, and salt.

3. In a medium bowl, lightly beat the eggs. Whisk in the vinegar, water, and oil. Stir in the nut pulp. Add the dry ingredients to the wet and mix until everything is completely incorporated.

4. FOR ROLLS: Divide the dough into 12 portions. Use your hands to roll each portion into a ball and place it on the parchment paper. If desired, sprinkle each with ¼ teaspoon sesame seeds and gently press down. Bake until the outside feels firm, 45 to 50 minutes.

FOR BUNS: Divide the dough into 4 to 6 portions depending on what size you want. Roll each portion into a ball. Place the balls on the parchment paper. Place a second sheet of parchment paper over the top of the balls. Use a cutting board to

recipe continues

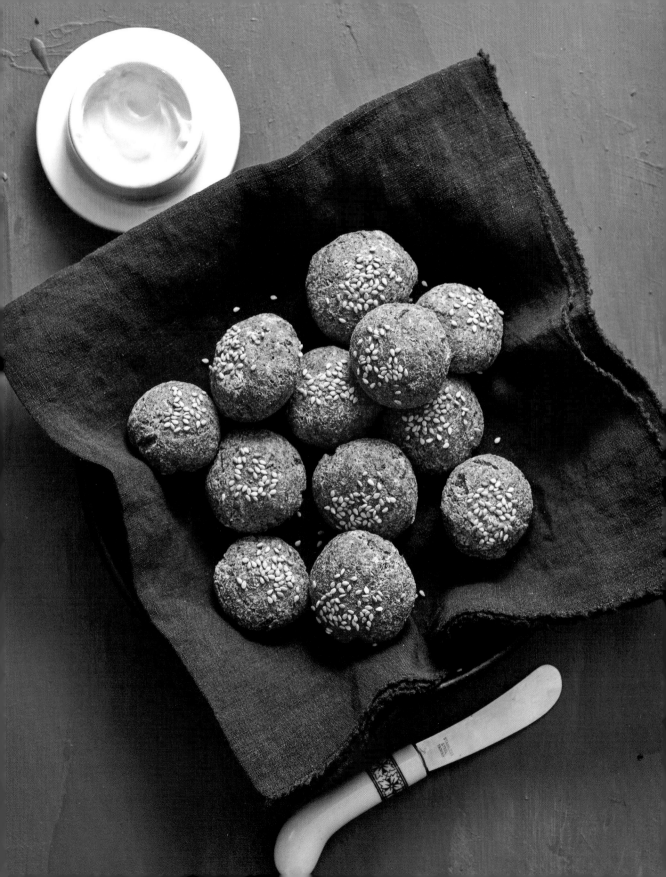

| MACRONUTRIENTS (PER ROLL) |
| CALORIES: 80 |
| FAT: 7 G/63 CALORIES |
| CARBOHYDRATE: 3 G/ 12 CALORIES |
| PROTEIN: 2 G/8 CALORIES |

| MACRONUTRIENTS (PER BUN) |
| CALORIES: 240 |
| FAT: 22 G/198 CALORIES |
| CARBOHYDRATE: 8 G/ 32 CALORIES |
| PROTEIN: 5 G/20 CALORIES |

press down until the buns are a little less than ½ inch thick. (Alternatively, cover with the second sheet of parchment and use a rolling pin to roll them out one at a time.) If desired, sprinkle with the sesame seeds and press down gently so they stick. Bake for 20 minutes, then flip and bake until they feel firm when you press down on them, another 5 to 10 minutes.

5. Allow the rolls or buns to cool for 5 to 10 minutes before serving. Store leftovers in an airtight container in the refrigerator.

COCONUT-ALMOND BITES

You'll notice that the flavors of these bites remind you of a candy bar that shall not be named, but without being such a massive sugar bomb.

MAKES 12 BITES

1 (3.5-ounce/100 g) bar dark chocolate (85% cacao or higher)

4 tablespoons coconut oil, melted

¼ cup unsweetened finely shredded coconut

¼ teaspoon stevia powder or keto-friendly sweetener of choice (optional)

¼ to ½ teaspoon flaky sea salt, such as Maldon

12 almonds

MACRONUTRIENTS PER BITE

CALORIES: 94

FAT: 9 G/81 CALORIES

CARBOHYDRATE: 4 G/
16 CALORIES

PROTEIN: 1 G/4 CALORIES

1. Break the chocolate bar into small chunks. Place the chocolate in a microwave-safe bowl, along with 2 tablespoons of the coconut oil. Microwave for 30 seconds. Stir. Continue to microwave in 10-second increments, stirring after each, until the chocolate is fully melted.

2. Divide the chocolate evenly among 12 cups of a silicone mini-muffin mold. Refrigerate for 5 minutes to harden.

3. Meanwhile, in a bowl, combine the remaining 2 tablespoons melted coconut oil, shredded coconut, and stevia (if using). Remove the chocolate from the refrigerator. Place about 1 teaspoon of the coconut mixture on top of each portion of chocolate, smoothing to cover. Sprinkle the bites with the flaky salt. Press 1 almond into the top of each. Place the bites in the freezer for at least 30 minutes to harden.

4. Remove the bites from the mold and store in an airtight container in the freezer. Serve straight from the freezer, allowing a couple minutes to sit at room temperature if frozen solid.

BERRY BLINTZES

Is this a treat or a breakfast food? It's really an any-time-of-day food that will please keto and non-keto folks alike.

SERVES 6

FOR THE BATTER

4 tablespoons (½ stick) unsalted butter, melted

4 large eggs

4 ounces full-fat cream cheese

2 tablespoons full-fat sour cream

½ cup full-fat coconut milk

1 teaspoon vanilla extract

½ cup coconut flour

¼ teaspoon ground cinnamon

FOR THE FILLING

2 large eggs

½ cup whole-milk ricotta cheese

½ cup coconut cream (see Note)

1 teaspoon vanilla extract

2 teaspoons grated lemon zest (preferably Meyer lemon)

1 teaspoon fresh lemon juice (preferably Meyer lemon)

Pinch of sea salt

1 cup frozen mixed berries, thawed

1. Preheat the oven to 350°F. Grease an 8 × 8-inch glass baking dish with 1 tablespoon of the melted butter.

2. For the batter: In a blender, combine the remaining 3 tablespoons melted butter, eggs, cream cheese, sour cream, coconut milk, vanilla, coconut flour, and cinnamon and blend until smooth.

3. Spoon half the batter into the greased baking dish and bake for 10 minutes.

4. Meanwhile, for the filling: In a small bowl, lightly beat the eggs, then mix in the ricotta and coconut cream. (If the cream is very thick, heat it in the microwave for 15 to 20 seconds to soften.) Stir in the vanilla, lemon zest, lemon juice, salt, and berries.

5. Remove the pan from the oven. Pour the filling over the baked egg batter and spread it out evenly. Return the pan to the oven and bake another 10 minutes.

6. Remove the pan from the oven. Drop the remaining egg batter over the filling by the spoonful, making an effort to cover most of the filling. (If some of the filling remains uncovered, that's fine.) Gently smooth over the top. Return the pan to the oven and bake until the filling and batter are totally set, another 20 minutes. Remove the pan from the oven and let stand for 10 minutes.

7. Use a sharp knife to cut the blintzes into 6 equal portions. Use a spatula to carefully remove them from the pan. Top with the optional toppings if desired and serve warm.

Note: For the coconut cream, you can purchase coconut cream, or you can carefully open a can of full-fat coconut milk and scoop the thick cream off the top.

TOPPINGS (OPTIONAL)

Unsalted butter

Coconut butter

Shredded coconut

Whipped cream made with heavy whipping cream (see page 239) or coconut milk

Ground cinnamon

MACRONUTRIENTS PER SERVING
(WITHOUT OPTIONAL TOPPINGS)

CALORIES: 349

FAT: 28 G/249 CALORIES

CARBOHYDRATE: 12 G/
48 CALORIES

PROTEIN: 12 G/50 CALORIES

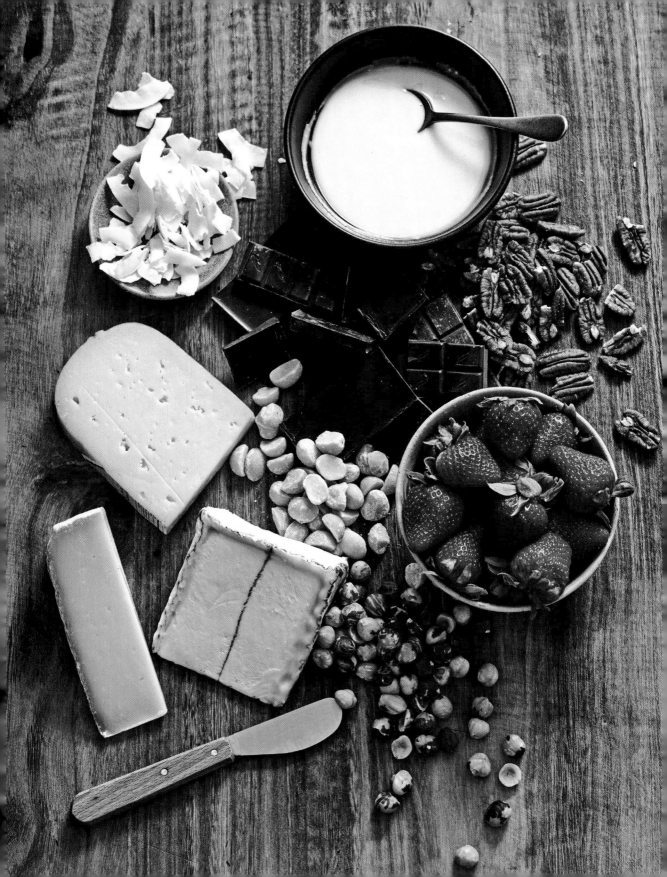

KETO ENTERTAINING PLATTER

There is really no need whatsoever to contemplate "keto treats," or to stress about what to serve non-keto guests, when you can put together this incredibly simple but elegant option in mere minutes.

SERVES 12
GENEROUSLY

3   (approximately 2.5- to 3.5-ounce) bars dark chocolate (85% cacao or higher), choose a variety

3   (4-ounce) wedges cheese, different varieties

¼   cup coconut butter

1   pint fresh berries, any type

½   cup large coconut flakes

½   cup macadamia nuts

½   cup pecans

½   cup hazelnuts

Select a large platter. Break the chocolate bars into bite-size pieces and arrange in three piles around the platter. Slice the cheese and arrange it in three piles on the platter. Place the coconut butter in a small ramekin and place it on the platter with a demitasse spoon for serving as a garnish. The berries, coconut flakes, and nuts can be placed in individual ramekins or simply arranged on the platter amid the chocolate and cheese.

MACRONUTRIENTS PER SERVING

CALORIES: 433

FAT: 39 G/347 CALORIES

CARBOHYDRATE: 11 G/
45 CALORIES

PROTEIN: 14 G/58 CALORIES

DAIRY-FREE AVOCADO MOUSSE

One of the popular recipes from *The Keto Reset Diet* is the rich avocado mousse made with a cream cheese base, but the dairy-free members of the Keto Reset community couldn't get in on the action. This dairy-free version draws on the flavors of Mexican chocolate and is every bit as good as the cream cheese version.

SERVES 2

2	ounces dark chocolate (see Note)
¼ to ½	cup coconut cream (see Note, page 229)
½	teaspoon vanilla extract
½	teaspoon ground cinnamon
⅛	teaspoon finely ground Himalayan sea salt
	Pinch of cayenne pepper, or more to taste
1	avocado
2 to 4	drops liquid stevia, or keto-friendly sweetener of choice (optional)
¼	teaspoon flaky sea salt, such as Maldon (optional)

1. Break the dark chocolate into chunks and place it in a microwave-safe bowl along with ¼ cup coconut cream. Microwave on high in 15-second increments, stirring after each, until the chocolate is melted.

2. Stir the vanilla, cinnamon, fine sea salt, and cayenne into the chocolate. Add the avocado and use a fork or, preferably, an immersion blender to mix in the avocado until smooth. Add more coconut cream as needed to achieve the desired consistency. Taste and add a sweetener if desired.

3. Divide the mousse between two ramekins. If desired, sprinkle with flaky salt. Eat it immediately, or cover and refrigerate the mousse until ready to serve.

Note: The darker the better when it comes to the chocolate in this recipe! Go as dark as possible with the 100% cacao Montezuma's Absolute Black bar (it can be found at Trader Joe's in the US and online), or the 100% cacao Fruition bar (Fruition.com).

MACRONUTRIENTS PER SERVING*

CALORIES: 334

FAT: 30 G/270 CALORIES

CARBOHYDRATE: 15 G/ 58 CALORIES

PROTEIN: 5 G/20 CALORIES

* Macros based on using ½ cup coconut cream.

CHAI PANNA COTTA

Panna cotta is an Italian custard. Enjoy this simple, dairy-free version that highlights the natural sweetness of coconut milk. Dress it up by topping it with coconut milk whipped cream (see *The Keto Reset Diet*) and pomegranate seeds.

SERVES 4

1½ cups full-fat coconut milk

1 teaspoon vanilla extract

1½ teaspoons chai spice blend, homemade (page 253) or store-bought

Pinch of Himalayan sea salt

5 to 10 drops liquid stevia (optional)

1½ teaspoons unflavored gelatin

MACRONUTRIENTS PER SERVING

CALORIES: 33

FAT: 2 G/18 CALORIES

CARBOHYDRATE: 3 G/ 12 CALORIES

PROTEIN: 1 G/4 CALORIES

1. In a medium saucepan, stir together the coconut milk, vanilla, spice blend, and salt. Taste the mixture and, if desired, sweeten with the stevia to taste.

2. Sprinkle the gelatin over the surface of the coconut milk. Allow it to sit for 5 minutes.

3. Place the saucepan over medium-low heat. Stir the gelatin into the coconut milk and continue to whisk regularly as the coconut milk warms. When the mixture begins to steam, and bubbles just appear around the edges, remove it from the heat. Give the mixture another good stir.

4. Pour the mixture evenly into four individual 3-inch rame-kins. Refrigerate for at least 2 hours to set. Serve cold.

Mix it up! Substitute pumpkin pie spice (see page 254) for the chai spice blend for a different flavor.

DARK CHOCOLATE PUDDING

This recipe was inspired by the pudding recipe from Samin Nosrat's incredible book *Salt Fat Acid Heat,* which is an excellent read for anyone who truly loves cooking. However, many of the recipes it contains aren't exactly keto. This take on Nosrat's chocolate pudding uses tapioca starch, erythritol, and heavy whipping cream to take the place of ingredients that are not keto-friendly. The final product is every bit the comfort food you expect homemade pudding to be.

SERVES 4

2.5 ounces dark chocolate (85% cacao or higher), broken into pieces

2 large eggs

2 tablespoons unsweetened cocoa powder

2 tablespoons tapioca starch

1 tablespoon erythritol, or other keto-friendly sweetener of choice

1 teaspoon kosher salt

½ teaspoon ground cinnamon

¼ teaspoon ground cardamom

1 cup heavy whipping cream

1 cup filtered water

MACRONUTRIENTS PER SERVING

CALORIES: 334

FAT: 29 G/261 CALORIES

CARBOHYDRATE: 18 G/ 72 CALORIES

PROTEIN: 6 G/24 CALORIES

1. Place the chocolate in a medium heatproof bowl and set a small fine-mesh sieve over the bowl. Set aside. In a medium heatproof bowl, lightly beat the eggs. Set aside.

2. In a small bowl, stir together the cocoa powder, tapioca starch, erythritol, salt, cinnamon, and cardamom. Set near the stove.

3. In a small saucepan, combine the cream and water and heat it over low heat, stirring regularly. As soon the first bubbles appear, whisk in the dry ingredients. Increase the heat to medium-low and cook the mixture for 3 minutes, stirring constantly. The mixture should become thick.

4. *Slowly* pour about half the pudding mixture into the eggs, stirring constantly to temper them. Stir this mixture back into the saucepan. Place the saucepan back over low heat and cook another 3 minutes, stirring constantly. Remove from the heat.

5. Pour the hot mixture through the sieve into the bowl with the chocolate. Use a large spoon or a spatula to push the cream mixture through the sieve. Stir the cream mixture into the chocolate until the chocolate is melted, then use an immersion blender to mix the pudding until it is very smooth.

6. Divide the mixture evenly among four individual serving cups. Allow the pudding to sit for about 30 minutes to come to room temperature before serving. Refrigerate any leftovers with a piece of plastic wrap covering the surface.

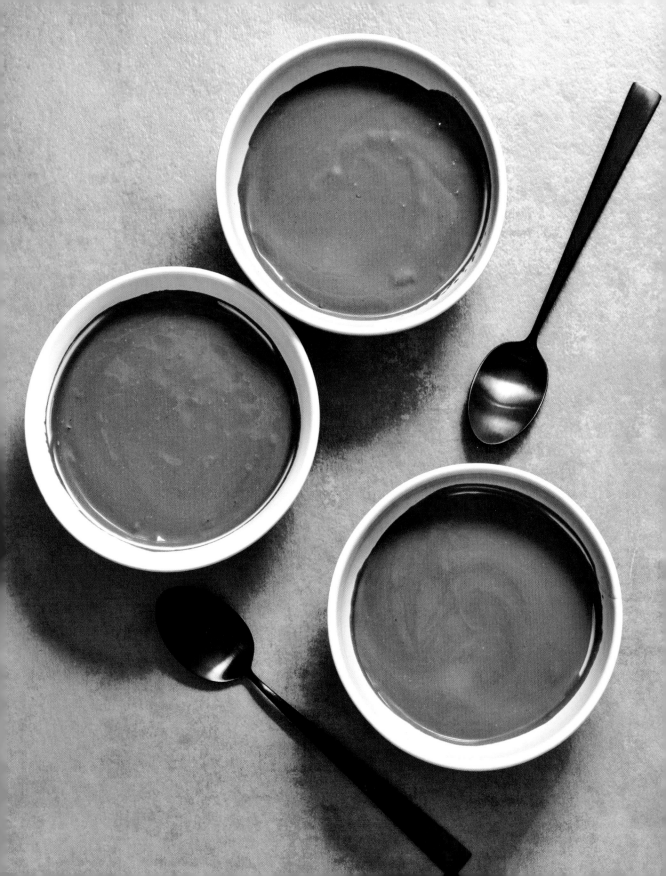

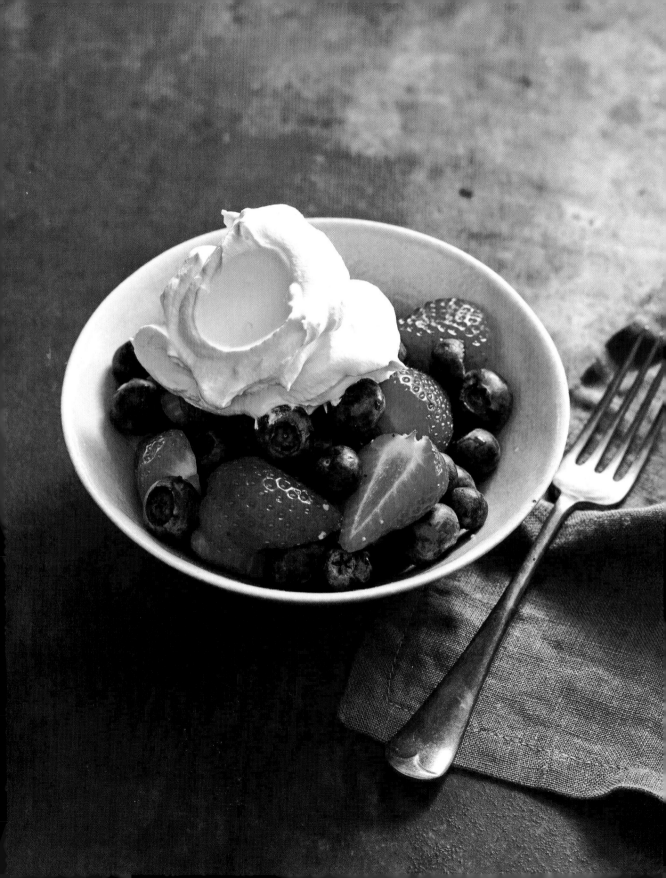

BERRIES WITH TANGY WHIP

One thing you'll notice after you switch to a primal or keto eating style is that the go-to treats from your "old life" suddenly taste unpleasantly sweet. This is a good thing! You learn to enjoy less-sweetened desserts, like these berries with sour cream whipped cream. Start with only a little (or even no!) sweetener and dial up the sweetness slowly to the minimum you find enjoyable. See if it changes over time.

SERVES 4

½ cup heavy whipping cream

¼ cup full-fat sour cream (see Note)

½ teaspoon vanilla extract

1 teaspoon grated lemon zest

1 teaspoon fresh lemon juice

5 drops liquid stevia, or to taste, or keto-friendly sweetener of choice (optional)

2 cups berries (any type), fresh or thawed frozen

1. Place the beaters from your mixer and a glass or metal bowl in the freezer for 30 minutes.

2. Remove the bowl from the freezer. Ideally, nest it inside a second larger bowl filled with ice cubes. Place the cream, sour cream, and vanilla in the chilled bowl.

3. Place the chilled beaters on your hand mixer and beat the cream mixture until it is light and fluffy. Add the lemon zest and lemon juice and beat for another few seconds. Taste it and decide if you are going to sweeten it or not. If yes, add the sweetener and beat for 5 seconds more.

4. Divide the berries among four individual ramekins. Top with the whipped cream and serve immediately.

Note: Instead of sour cream, you can substitute crème fraîche, full-fat Greek yogurt, or full-fat coconut milk yogurt.

MACRONUTRIENTS PER SERVING

CALORIES: 71

FAT: 3 G/27 CALORIES

CARBOHYDRATE: 10 G/ 40 CALORIES

PROTEIN: 1 G/4 CALORIES

KEY LIME PISTACHIO MUG CAKE

I make this whenever I can find key limes in the store (which is much easier since my move to Miami!), but regular limes will do in a pinch. Key limes have a special flavor, though, so use them if you can.

SERVES 1

- 1 tablespoon salted butter
- ½ teaspoon grated key lime or regular lime zest
- 1 teaspoon key lime or regular lime juice
- ¼ teaspoon vanilla extract
- 1 teaspoon monkfruit sweetener or keto-friendly sweetener of choice
- 2 tablespoons blanched almond flour

  Scant ¼ teaspoon baking soda

  Pinch of sea salt

- 1 large egg, at room temperature
- 2 teaspoons crushed raw or dry-roasted pistachios

1. Place the butter in a mug. Microwave for 20 seconds. Stir.

2. Stir in the lime zest, lime juice, vanilla, and sweetener. Add the almond flour, baking soda, and salt, and stir again. Add the egg and mix well until completely incorporated.

3. Sprinkle the pistachios over the top and stir just once. You want them to stay near the top of the batter.

4. Microwave on high for 1 minute. Remove from the micro-wave and let sit for 2 minutes. Enjoy warm.

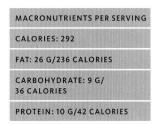

MACRONUTRIENTS PER SERVING

CALORIES: 292

FAT: 26 G/236 CALORIES

CARBOHYDRATE: 9 G/ 36 CALORIES

PROTEIN: 10 G/42 CALORIES

WHIPPED CREAM

Your basic keto whipped cream!

MAKES ABOUT
2 CUPS

½ pint heavy whipping cream

1 teaspoon vanilla extract

2 to 3 drops liquid stevia (optional)

MACRONUTRIENTS PER ¼ CUP
CALORIES: 176
FAT: 19 G/167 CALORIES
CARBOHYDRATE: 2 G/ 7 CALORIES
PROTEIN: 1 G/5 CALORIES

1. Place the beaters from your mixer and a glass or metal bowl in the freezer for 30 minutes.

2. Remove the bowl from the freezer. Ideally, nest it inside a second larger bowl filled with ice cubes. Place the cream and vanilla in the chilled bowl.

3. Place the chilled beaters on your hand mixer and beat the cream mixture until it is light and fluffy. Taste it and decide if you are going to sweeten it or not. If yes, add the sweetener and beat for 5 seconds more. Use immediately.

BEVERAGES

KETO RESET COFFEE

This version goes above and beyond your basic high-fat coffee (which is often criticized as being less nutritious than a high-fat meal such as an omelet) with the introduction of special ingredients—a raw egg, medium chain triglyceride (MCT) oil, and collagen protein powder. The egg yolk provides an assortment of important micronutrients like choline; the MCT oil is a catalyst for ketone production in the liver; and the collagen peptides boost the health of joints and connective tissue in areas where you need support the most. More than just a morning fat bomb, wouldn't you say?

SERVES 1

- 1 large egg
- 1 tablespoon MCT oil
- 1 tablespoon heavy whipping cream or full-fat coconut milk
- ¼ teaspoon ground cinnamon
- 1 cup freshly brewed coffee
- 2 heaping tablespoons collagen peptides or hydrolysate

1. Place the egg, MCT oil, cream, and cinnamon in a jar with a mouth wide enough to fit your immersion blender. (If you do not have an immersion blender, you can use a regular blender, but an immersion blender is ideal.) Blend until frothy.

2. With the blender running, slowly pour in the coffee. If you add it too fast, the egg will scramble.

3. Pour the coffee mixture into a mug and stir in the collagen peptides. Enjoy immediately.

MACRONUTRIENTS PER SERVING

CALORIES: 291

FAT: 24 G/217 CALORIES

CARBOHYDRATE: 3 G/ 10 CALORIES

PROTEIN: 17 G/68 CALORIES

KETO COLLAGEN GREEN TEA LATTE

This latte is so good that it might just turn the most devoted coffee lover into a tea drinker! If you are trying to get extra healthy fats or want the ketone-boosting effects of MCT oil, include it in the recipe; but if you would rather eat your fats with whole foods, feel free to omit it.

SERVES 1

- 1 bag green tea of your choice
- 1 cup boiling water
- ½ teaspoon matcha powder
- 2 tablespoons coconut cream (see Note, page 229)
- 1 tablespoon MCT oil (optional)
- 1 scoop vanilla-flavored collagen powder or whey protein (see Note)

1. Steep the tea bag in the just-boiled water for 3 minutes. Remove.

2. Pour the tea into a jar with a mouth wide enough to fit your immersion blender. (If you do not have an immersion blender, you can use a regular blender.) Add the matcha powder, coconut cream, and MCT oil (if using). Blend for 15 seconds. Pour into a mug and stir in the collagen powder. Enjoy hot.

Note: Choose *either* whey protein or collagen powder (peptides or hydrolysate), not both, because collagen protein is best assimilated by itself, without other proteins. Primal Kitchen Vanilla Coconut Collagen Fuel is my go-to flavor for this recipe. If you use unflavored collagen powder, add ¼ teaspoon vanilla extract and 2 to 3 drops liquid stevia.

MACRONUTRIENTS PER SERVING* (NO MCT OIL)
CALORIES: 124
FAT: 7 G/66 CALORIES
CARBOHYDRATE: 4 G/16 CALORIES
PROTEIN: 11 G/45 CALORIES
* Macros based on using Primal Kitchen Vanilla Coconut Collagen Fuel.

MACRONUTRIENTS PER SERVING* (WITH MCT OIL)
CALORIES: 249
FAT: 21 G/192 CALORIES
CARBOHYDRATE: 4 G/16 CALORIES
PROTEIN: 11 G/45 CALORIES
* Macros based on using Primal Kitchen Vanilla Coconut Collagen Fuel.

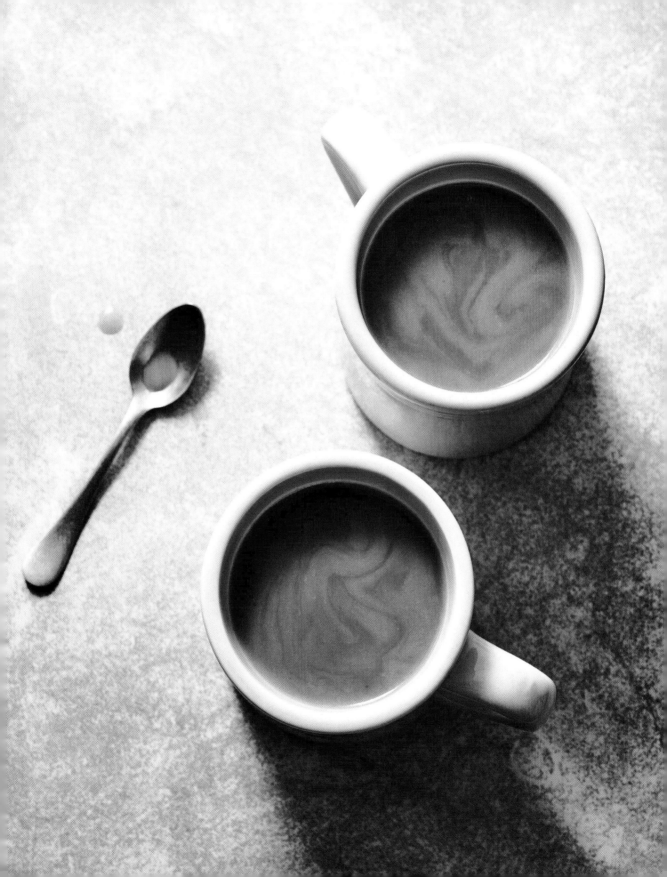

PUMPKIN SPICE LATTE

Yes, you can enjoy pumpkin on a keto diet! However, you're going to find it impossible to find a pumpkin spice latte—the official drink of fall—in a traditional coffee shop or store-bought container that isn't loaded with sugar. No worries, this recipe has you covered. If you enjoy the ketone-boosting effects of MCT oil, use it here, or feel free to omit it.

SERVES 2

3   tablespoons Homemade Pumpkin Puree (recipe follows) or unsweetened canned

2   tablespoons heavy whipping cream or full-fat coconut milk

¾   teaspoon Pumpkin Pie Spice Blend (page 254)

2   tablespoons MCT oil (optional)

2   cups freshly brewed coffee

1   scoop vanilla-flavored whey protein powder

1. In a blender, combine the pumpkin puree, cream, pumpkin pie spice, MCT oil (if using), and about ½ cup coffee and blend until smooth.

2. With the blender running, slowly pour in the rest of the coffee. Blend for about 10 seconds, until frothy. Add in the vanilla protein powder. Pulse a few times to combine.

3. Strain the mixture through a fine-mesh sieve. Pour into two mugs and enjoy hot.

MACRONUTRIENTS PER SERVING* (NO MCT OIL)
CALORIES: 113
FAT: 8 G/71 CALORIES
CARBOHYDRATE: 7 G/ 29 CALORIES
PROTEIN: 6 G/25 CALORIES
* Macros based on using Primal Fuel Vanilla Coconut Protein Powder.

MACRONUTRIENTS PER SERVING* (WITH MCT OIL)
CALORIES: 238
FAT: 8 G/197 CALORIES
CARBOHYDRATE: 7 G/ 29 CALORIES
PROTEIN: 6 G/25 CALORIES
* Macros based on using Primal Fuel Vanilla Coconut Protein Powder.

HOMEMADE PUMPKIN PUREE

It is incredibly easy to make your own pumpkin puree, especially if you have an Instant Pot. Use your homemade pumpkin puree in Kale Salad with Pumpkin "Croutons" (page 92) and Keto Kaddo Bourani (page 158).

MAKES ABOUT 3 CUPS

1   small pie pumpkin (about 3 pounds)

MACRONUTRIENTS PER ¼ CUP
CALORIES: 20
FAT: 0 G/0 CALORIES
CARBOHYDRATE: 5 G/ 20 CALORIES
PROTEIN: <1 G/2 CALORIES

1. Use a sharp knife to carefully cut the pumpkin into quarters and scoop out the seeds and strings.

2. Pour 1 cup water into the Instant Pot. Place the metal steam rack/trivet inside. Arrange the pieces of pumpkin flesh side down on the rack (it is okay if they overlap). Secure the lid and set the steam release valve to Sealing. Press the Manual button and set the time for 20 minutes.

3. When the Instant Pot beeps, allow the pressure to release naturally. When fully released, carefully open the lid and remove the pumpkin. The flesh should easily separate from the skin.

4. Discard the skin and use a potato masher or blender to puree the flesh. Store in an airtight container in the refrigerator. Freeze any puree you do not intend to use within a few days.

GARLICKY BONE BROTH

A hot mug of bone broth with just a little salt is the ultimate in comfort, but sometimes it is nice to mix it up, too. This is an easy way to do something different and keep vampires at bay at the same time. Win-win!

SERVES 1

2 tablespoons unsalted butter or ghee

3 large cloves garlic, chopped

1½ cups chicken or beef bone broth, homemade (page 35) or store-bought

Sea salt and ground black pepper

1. In a medium saucepan, melt the butter over medium heat. Add the garlic and sauté until the garlic is just soft, about 2 minutes.

2. Add the broth and heat just until hot. Remove it from the heat. Use an immersion blender (or a traditional blender) to carefully blend it until smooth. Season with salt and pepper to taste. Drink hot.

MACRONUTRIENTS PER SERVING

CALORIES: 291

FAT: 27 G/247 CALORIES

CARBOHYDRATE: 3 G/ 14 CALORIES

PROTEIN: 9 G/34 CALORIES

GOLDEN BONE BROTH

This recipe packs so many health punches—the many gut-healing and immune-supporting benefits of collagen-rich bone broth, combined with the anti-inflammatory super-spice turmeric. When cooking with turmeric, always pair it with black pepper. This makes the primary bioactive component of turmeric, called curcumin, more bioavailable.

SERVES 1

1 to 2   tablespoons ghee or coconut oil

½   teaspoon ground turmeric

¼   teaspoon ground cinnamon

¼   teaspoon ground ginger

Ground black pepper

1½   cups chicken bone broth, homemade (page 35) or store-bought

Sea salt

1. In a small saucepan, melt the ghee over low heat. Add the turmeric, cinnamon, ginger, and ¼ teaspoon pepper and sauté until fragrant, 15 to 30 seconds.

2. Add the broth and increase the heat to medium. Heat until a few bubbles appear. Remove it from the heat. Use an immersion blender (or a regular blender) to carefully blend the broth until frothy. Do not skip the blending step, otherwise the ghee will just float on the surface. Season with salt and more pepper to taste. Drink hot.

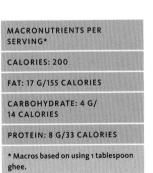

MACRONUTRIENTS PER SERVING*

CALORIES: 200

FAT: 17 G/155 CALORIES

CARBOHYDRATE: 4 G/ 14 CALORIES

PROTEIN: 8 G/33 CALORIES

* Macros based on using 1 tablespoon ghee.

CREAMY KETO HOT CHOCOLATE (DAIRY-FREE)

We all know how hot chocolate hits the spot during the colder months, and what a cultural centerpiece it occupies, but have you ever examined a label of the instant packets or even a "gourmet" powdered cocoa product? Massive sugar bomb—no-go for keto! This keto-friendly version is just as satisfying, and you get a dose of healthy fats and collagen for joint and skin health. You can cut the amount of cacao butter in half if you want; it will still be delicious, just a little less creamy.

SERVES 1

- 1 cup Nut Milk (page 38), or full-fat coconut milk
- 1 tablespoon raw cacao butter
- 1/8 teaspoon peppermint extract (optional)
- 1 scoop chocolate-flavored collagen powder or whey protein (see Note, page 242)

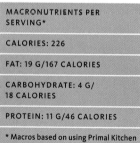

MACRONUTRIENTS PER SERVING*

CALORIES: 226

FAT: 19 G/167 CALORIES

CARBOHYDRATE: 4 G/ 18 CALORIES

PROTEIN: 11 G/46 CALORIES

* Macros based on using Primal Kitchen Chocolate Coconut Collagen Fuel.

1. In a small saucepan, combine the nut milk, cacao butter, and peppermint extract (if using) and heat over medium-low to medium heat until the cacao butter is melted. Remove it from the heat. Use an immersion blender (or regular blender) to carefully blend on high speed until frothy, 15 to 20 seconds.

2. Stir in the collagen powder, or pulse it a few times on low speed with the blender. Pour it into a mug and enjoy hot.

Mix it up! Replace half the nut milk with coffee—or espresso if you're feeling fancy!—for a collagen mocha (with or without the peppermint extract). Top the hot chocolate with fresh Whipped Cream (page 239) or coconut milk whipped cream (which you can find in the *The Keto Reset Diet*) and a sprinkling of cinnamon.

KETO ITALIAN CREAM SODA

A traditional Italian soda is made with flavored (and sugar-packed) Torani syrup and club soda. Adding cream makes it a cream soda. This version has none of the sugar but all the creamy deliciousness. It is a great party "mocktail" or afternoon treat that delivers a bit of healthy fat.

SERVES 1

Ice

1 (12-ounce) can unsweetened sparkling mineral water, any flavor

2 drops liquid stevia (optional)

1 to 2 tablespoons heavy whipping cream (or full-fat coconut milk if dairy-free)

1. Fill a highball glass halfway with ice. Add the sparkling water to 1 inch from the top. If you are using stevia, add it and gently stir.

2. Slowly pour the heavy cream on top. Stir if desired, or let the cream slowly settle. This is best drunk with a straw.

MACRONUTRIENTS PER SERVING*
CALORIES: 102
FAT: 11 G/97 CALORIES
CARBOHYDRATE: 1 G/3 CALORIES
PROTEIN: 1 G/4 CALORIES
* Macros based on using 2 tablespoons cream.

Mix it up! Try one of these combinations:

- Lemon cream pie = lemon sparkling water + a squirt of fresh lemon juice + heavy whipping cream + stevia
- Piña colada = pineapple sparkling water + coconut milk

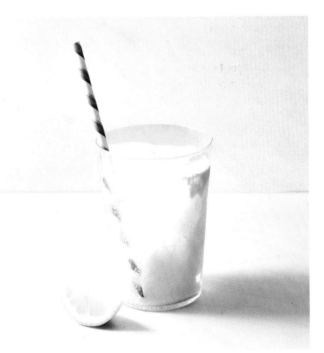

SPICE BLENDS

Spice blends are the easiest way to add an interesting dimension to basic ingredients and recipes. Since many commercially available blends contain cornstarch and/or sugar (look for dextrose, sucrose, or maltodextrin on the label), it is often better to make your own. You will notice that all but one of these recipes do not include salt. This allows you to control the salt within individual recipes.

For all of these recipes (except the Za'atar Seasoning on page 255), in a small bowl, stir together all the ingredients. Transfer to a small glass container. The best containers are old empty spice jars. For spice blends you use frequently, consider doubling or tripling the recipe.

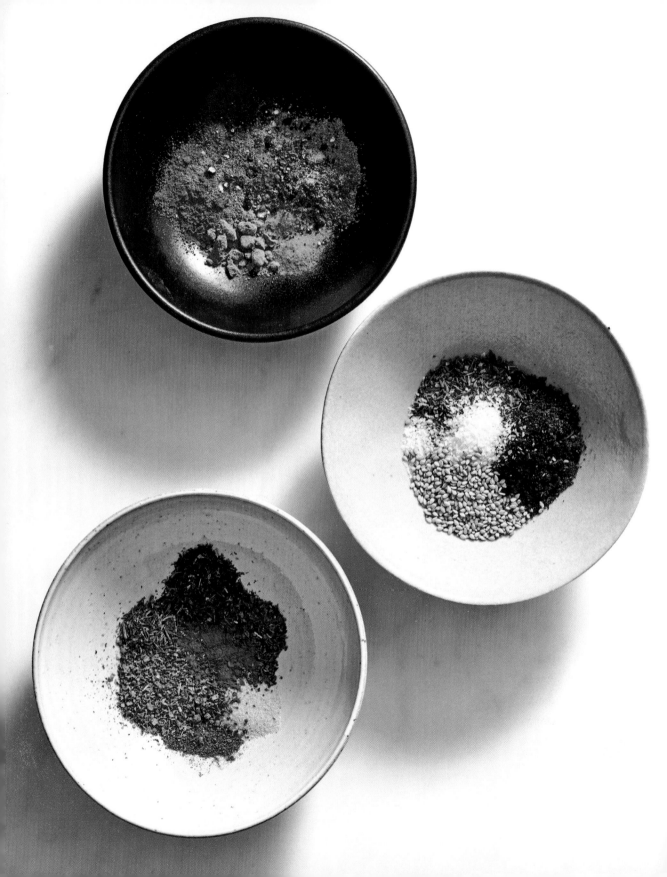

BAKING POWDER

- 2 tablespoons cream of tartar
- 2 tablespoons arrowroot powder
- 1 tablespoon baking soda

CAJUN SEASONING

- 2 tablespoons sweet paprika
- 1 tablespoon garlic powder
- 1 tablespoon onion powder
- 1 teaspoon dried oregano
- 1 teaspoon dried thyme
- ½ teaspoon ground black pepper
- ½ teaspoon ground white pepper (or additional black pepper)
- ⅛ to ¼ teaspoon cayenne pepper

CHAI SPICE BLEND

- 2 teaspoons ground cardamom
- 2 teaspoons ground cinnamon
- 1 teaspoon ground allspice
- 1 teaspoon ground cloves
- 1 teaspoon ground ginger

CHOCO-CHILI RUB

- 1 tablespoon chili powder
- 1 tablespoon unsweetened cocoa powder
- 1 teaspoon ground cumin
- 1 teaspoon smoked paprika
- ½ teaspoon dried oregano
- ½ teaspoon ground coriander
- ¼ teaspoon ground allspice
- ¼ teaspoon espresso powder (optional)

GREEK SEASONING BLEND

- 1 tablespoon dried basil
- 1 tablespoon dried oregano
- 1 tablespoon garlic powder
- 2 teaspoons onion powder
- 2 teaspoons ground black pepper
- 1 teaspoon dried dill
- 1 teaspoon dried marjoram
- ½ teaspoon dried thyme
- ½ teaspoon ground cinnamon
- ½ teaspoon ground nutmeg

ITALIAN SEASONING BLEND

- 1   tablespoon dried basil
- 1   tablespoon dried oregano
- 1   tablespoon dried marjoram
- 1   tablespoon dried parsley
- 1   teaspoon dried rosemary
- 1   teaspoon dried thyme
- 1   teaspoon garlic powder

JERK SEASONING BLEND

- 1   tablespoon garlic powder
- 2   teaspoons onion powder
- 2   teaspoons dried thyme
- 2   teaspoons dried parsley
- 1   teaspoon sweet paprika
- 1   teaspoon ground allspice
- ½   teaspoon cayenne pepper
- ½   teaspoon red pepper flakes
- ½   teaspoon ground black pepper
- ½   teaspoon ground nutmeg
- ¼   teaspoon ground cinnamon
- ¼   teaspoon ground cumin

Note: If you like your jerk spicy, increase the amount of cayenne pepper!

PUMPKIN PIE SPICE BLEND

- 2   tablespoons ground cinnamon
- 1   teaspoon ground ginger
- 1   teaspoon ground nutmeg
- ½   teaspoon ground cloves
- ¼   teaspoon ground allspice

RAS EL HANOUT

- 2   teaspoons ground coriander
- 2   teaspoons ground cumin
- 1   teaspoon ground cinnamon
- 1   teaspoon ground turmeric
- ½   teaspoon ground allspice
- ½   teaspoon ground ginger
- ½   teaspoon sweet paprika
- ¼   teaspoon ground cloves
- ¼   teaspoon ground nutmeg
- ¼   teaspoon ground black pepper
- ⅛   teaspoon cayenne pepper (optional)

TACO SEASONING BLEND

- 1 tablespoon chili powder
- 1½ teaspoons ground cumin
- ½ teaspoon smoked paprika
- ¼ teaspoon dried oregano
- ¼ teaspoon red pepper flakes (optional)
- ¼ teaspoon garlic powder
- ¼ teaspoon onion powder

ZA'ATAR SEASONING

- 1 tablespoon ground sumac
- 1 tablespoon dried thyme
- 1 tablespoon toasted sesame seeds
- 1 teaspoon kosher salt

Combine all the ingredients in a mortar and pestle or spice grinder. Grind until the sesame seeds are crushed and blended with the other ingredients. Store in an airtight jar.

SAUCES & CONDIMENTS

QUICK HOLLANDAISE

Hollandaise is a great addition to a keto diet, and this easy recipe lets you whip up a batch in less than two minutes. Be sure to use unsalted butter in the preparation and then adjust the saltiness of the final product to taste.

MAKES A GENEROUS ³/₄ CUP

½ cup unsalted butter

3 egg yolks, at room temperature

Scant 1 tablespoon fresh lemon juice

Pinch of sea salt

Pinch of ground black pepper

⅛ teaspoon Cajun Seasoning (optional; page 253)

Keto-friendly hot sauce (optional)

MACRONUTRIENTS PER 2 TABLESPOONS
CALORIES: 163
FAT: 18 G/158 CALORIES
CARBOHYDRATE: <1 G/ 2 CALORIES
PROTEIN: 2 G/6 CALORIES

1. Place the butter in a microwave-safe glass container, ideally a small measuring cup with a spout. Microwave on high for 30 to 45 seconds to just melt.

2. In a jar with a mouth wide enough to fit your immersion blender, combine the egg yolks, lemon juice, salt, pepper, and Cajun seasoning (if using). Blend about 10 seconds to combine.

3. Give the melted butter a stir. With the immersion blender running in the egg yolk mixture, add the butter in a steady stream. Try to lift the immersion blender and move it around a bit to let the butter fully incorporate. Blend a few more seconds to make sure everything is fully blended.

4. Taste your hollandaise and adjust the seasoning. If desired, stir in hot sauce to taste. Use immediately or store in the refrigerator. This hollandaise keeps for several days, just give it a stir when you take it out of the fridge.

KETO "BBQ SAUCE"

This sauce doesn't taste like most BBQ sauces out there because it isn't sweetened. You will quickly habituate to its rich flavor, and store-bought stuff will taste too sweet. If you want to punch it up a bit, you can add a dash of honey or other sweetener, but this one works hard to be a flavorful alternative to sweet sauces.

**MAKES ABOUT
1 CUP**

¾ cup chicken bone broth, homemade (page 35) or store-bought, or vegetable stock

3 tablespoons tomato paste

1½ tablespoons apple cider vinegar

1½ tablespoons Dijon mustard

1½ teaspoons fish sauce

1½ teaspoons coconut aminos or tamari

½ teaspoon garlic powder

½ teaspoon onion powder

½ teaspoon chili powder

Heaping ¼ teaspoon sea salt

¼ teaspoon ground cinnamon

In a small saucepan, combine all the ingredients and bring to a boil. Reduce the heat to a simmer and simmer for 15 minutes to thicken and meld the flavors. Taste and adjust the salt. Use immediately, or store in an airtight container in the refrigerator for up to 4 days.

MACRONUTRIENTS PER ¼ CUP

CALORIES: 29

FAT: 1 G/7 CALORIES

CARBOHYDRATE: 4 G/ 16 CALORIES

PROTEIN: 2 G/8 CALORIES

TAHINI DRESSING OR DIPPING SAUCE

Tahini is a paste made from sesame seeds. It is a delicious alternative to nut butters in creamy sauces and dressings. Use this sauce as a dipping sauce for meats or vegetables, or thin it out with warm water and use it as a salad dressing.

MAKES ABOUT 1 CUP

¼ cup tahini

¼ cup extra-virgin olive oil

2 tablespoons tamari

2 tablespoons fresh lemon juice or lime juice

1 clove garlic, pressed or finely minced

¼ teaspoon ground cumin

¼ teaspoon ground ginger

Warm water

Sea salt

1. In a high-powered blender or food processor, combine the tahini, olive oil, tamari, lemon juice, garlic, cumin, and ginger and blend until smooth.

2. Stop the blender and use a spatula to scrape down the sides. With the blender running, slowly add warm water until the mixture reaches the desired consistency. Taste and add salt if desired. Store in the refrigerator in an airtight container. Use within 1 week.

MACRONUTRIENTS PER ¼ CUP

CALORIES: 217

FAT: 22 G/194 CALORIES

CARBOHYDRATE: 5 G/ 18 CALORIES

PROTEIN: 3 G/14 CALORIES

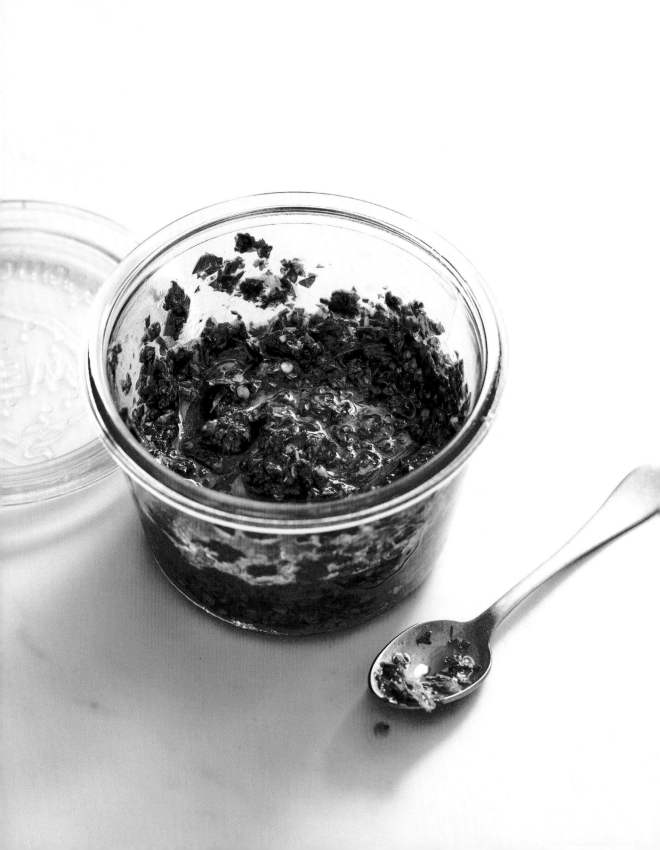

CHIMICHURRI

Chimichurri is a South American sauce and marinade. Traditionally made with parsley, oregano, garlic, red wine vinegar, and olive oil, it is a tasty and easy way to add flavor and healthy fat to your meals. It pairs well with most any meat or vegetable, and is especially delicious set against the smoky flavor of grilled meats or kebabs. Try it on scrambled eggs or sardines, too!

MAKES ABOUT 1½ CUPS

- 1 cup packed fresh flat-leaf parsley leaves
- 1 cup packed fresh cilantro leaves
- 4 medium cloves garlic, smashed
- 1 tablespoon dried oregano
- ¼ cup red wine vinegar
- ½ teaspoon kosher salt
- ¼ teaspoon ground black pepper
- ¼ to ½ teaspoon red pepper flakes (optional)
- 1 cup extra-virgin olive oil

1. In a high-powered blender or food processor, combine the fresh herbs, garlic, oregano, vinegar, salt, black pepper, pepper flakes (if using), and ¼ cup of the olive oil. Blend until the herbs are well chopped, 20 to 30 seconds. Stop the blender and use a spatula to scrape down the sides.

2. With the blender running, slowly pour in the remaining ¾ cup olive oil (or a little less if you want a thicker sauce). Transfer the chimichurri to a jar and store in the refrigerator. Use within 1 week.

MACRONUTRIENTS PER ¼ CUP
CALORIES: 329
FAT: 36 G/325 CALORIES
CARBOHYDRATE: 2 G/ 7 CALORIES
PROTEIN: 1 G/2 CALORIES

AIOLI

Aioli is basically a fancy name for garlic mayo. The food police will tell you that aioli should be made with a mortar and pestle and must include olive oil, so this one, which uses an avocado oil–based mayo and neither a mortar nor a pestle, is not *technically* a proper aioli. It can be our secret.

MAKES A GENEROUS ¹/₂ CUP

½ cup avocado oil mayonnaise

2 cloves garlic, pressed or very finely minced

2 teaspoons Dijon mustard

2 teaspoons fresh lemon juice, or to taste

Pinch of ground black pepper

Pinch of cayenne pepper

Whisk all the ingredients together. Store in the refrigerator in an airtight container. Use within 1 week.

Mix it up! Substitute Primal Kitchen Chipotle Lime Mayo (and omit the Dijon mustard) for an interesting twist.

MACRONUTRIENTS PER 2 TABLESPOONS

CALORIES: 103

FAT: 11 G/100 CALORIES

CARBOHYDRATE: 1 G/ 2 CALORIES

PROTEIN: <1 G/<1 CALORIE

TARTAR SAUCE

When you think tartar sauce, you probably think fish and chips. Serve this tartar sauce with Crispy Baked Cod (page 156) or Tuna Cakes (page 147).

¾ cup avocado oil mayonnaise

3 tablespoons finely chopped dill pickle (about 1 medium)

2 scallions, finely chopped

1½ teaspoons very finely chopped fresh parsley

1 tablespoon fresh lemon juice

1½ teaspoons Dijon mustard

Dash of keto-friendly hot sauce (optional)

MACRONUTRIENTS PER ¼ CUP

CALORIES: 307

FAT: 33 G/298 CALORIES

CARBOHYDRATE: 1 G/ 5 CALORIES

PROTEIN: <1 G/1 CALORIE

Stir together all the ingredients in a bowl. Refrigerate to chill. If you are not going to use it within a few hours, transfer it to a jar. It will keep in the refrigerator for 1 week.

PRIMAL-CESTERSHIRE SAUCE

Worcestershire sauce is a common ingredient in dishes that need a bit of umami, but store-bought Worcestershire is neither primal- nor keto-friendly because it contains molasses and often other objectionable ingredients. Since several of the recipes in this book are improved by Worcestershire, I recommend that you whip up a batch of this condiment to have on hand instead.

MAKES A GENEROUS ¾ CUP

½ cup apple cider vinegar

¼ cup coconut aminos

1 tablespoon Dijon mustard

½ teaspoon onion powder

¼ teaspoon garlic powder

⅛ teaspoon ground cinnamon

MACRONUTRIENTS PER 1 TABLESPOON

CALORIES: 14

FAT: <1 G/1 CALORIE

CARBOHYDRATE: 2 G/ 9 CALORIES

PROTEIN: <1 G/<1 CALORIE

Place all the ingredients in a jar with a tight-fitting lid. Shake vigorously to combine. Store this sauce in the refrigerator. Before using, shake vigorously again.

BRAD'S PESTO

My *Keto Reset Diet* coauthor, Brad Kearns, is known for throwing ingredients together in the kitchen and whipping up delicious meals almost by accident. This pesto is featured in Brad's Scallops with Pesto (page 155), but it's fabulous on everything from eggs to spaghetti squash to roasted veggies to grilled chicken.

MAKES A GENEROUS 1 CUP

- 2 cups packed fresh basil leaves
- ¼ cup pine nuts
- 2 cloves garlic, smashed
- 1 tablespoon fresh lemon juice
- 1 tablespoon chopped sun-dried tomatoes packed in olive oil (optional)
- ½ cup extra-virgin olive oil

In a food processor, combine the basil, pine nuts, garlic, lemon juice, and sun-dried tomato (if using). Pulse until the mixture resembles coarse sand. Scrape down the sides of the food processor with a spatula, then add ¼ cup of the olive oil. Process the mixture until it is thoroughly combined. With the food processor running, slowly drizzle in the remaining ¼ cup olive oil. You want the pesto to be thick.

MACRONUTRIENTS PER ¼ CUP

CALORIES: 309

FAT: 32 G/291 CALORIES

CARBOHYDRATE: 5 G/ 19 CALORIES

PROTEIN: 2 G/7 CALORIES

WILD RANCH DRESSING

Whip up this quick, creamy dressing in a jiffy for dipping air-fried chicken wings, raw vegetables, or lettuce wraps like the Handheld Chef Salad (page 103).

MAKES ABOUT 1 CUP

½ cup avocado oil mayonnaise

½ cup full-fat coconut milk

¾ teaspoon dried dill

1 teaspoon minced fresh chives

¼ teaspoon onion powder

⅛ teaspoon ground black pepper

Pinch of sea salt

In a small bowl, mix together all ingredients by hand until smooth. Add more salt to taste if needed. Store in the refrigerator in an airtight container. Use within 1 week.

MACRONUTRIENTS PER ¼ CUP

CALORIES: 256

FAT: 28 G/248 CALORIES

CARBOHYDRATE: 1 G/3 CALORIES

PROTEIN: 1 G/2 CALORIES

INDEX

Note: Page references in *italics* indicate photographs.

ABOUT THE AUTHORS

MARK SISSON presides over a wide-ranging Primal enterprise featuring the wildly popular Primal Kitchen line of healthy condiments, the Primal Health Coach Institute, a line of premium performance and nutritional supplements, and numerous books and online educational courses. A former world-class athlete in the marathon and ironman triathlon, he is considered a founding father of the Primal/paleo/keto health movement. He publishes daily tips and inspiration at MarksDailyApple.com, the top-ranked blog in its category for more than a decade.

LINDSAY TAYLOR, PhD, writes and researches for Sisson's Primal Blueprint enterprise, hosting podcasts and serving as the lead moderator on the thriving Keto Reset and Primal Endurance communities on Facebook. Find her healthy, colorful meal creations on Instagram @theusefuldish.